APPLICATIONS MANUAL FOR

Health & Physical Assessment in Nursing

D'AMICO • BARBARITO

3rd EDITION

APPLICATIONS MANUAL FOR

Health & Physical Assessment in Nursing

D'AMICO • BARBARITO

3rd EDITION

Donita D'Amico, MEd, RN
Associate Professor
William Paterson University
Wayne, New Jersey

Colleen Barbarito, EdD, RN
Associate Professor
William Paterson University
Wayne, New Jersey

Contributing Editors
Christina D. Keller, RN, MSN
Instructor
Radford University School of Nursing and Clinical Simulation Center
Radford, Virginia

Laura R. Durbin, RN, MSN
Associate Professor
West Kentucky Community and Technical College
Paducah, Kentucky

PEARSON

Boston   Columbus   Indianapolis   New York   San Francisco
Amsterdam   Cape Town   Dubai   London   Madrid   Milan   Munich   Paris   Montreal   Toronto
Delhi   Mexico City   São Paulo   Sydney   Hong Kong   Seoul   Singapore   Taipei   Tokyo

Publisher: Julie Levin Alexander
Publisher's Assistant: Sarah Henrich
Executive Editor: Pamela Fuller
Development Editor: S4Carlisle Publishing Services
Editorial Assistant: Erin Sullivan
Project Manager: Cathy O'Connell
Program Manager: Erin Rafferty
Director, Product Management Services: Etain O'Dea
Team Lead, Program Management: Melissa Bashe
Team Lead, Project Management: Cynthia Zonneveld
Full-Service Project Manager: Kannan Poojali,
　S4Carlisle Publishing Services

Manufacturing Buyer: Maura Zaldivar-Garcia
Art Director: Maria Guglielmo
Vice President of Sales & Marketing: David Gesell
Vice President, Director of Marketing: Margaret Waples
Senior Product Marketing Manager: Phoenix Harvey
Field Marketing Manager: Debi Doyle
Marketing Specialist: Michael Sirinides
Marketing Assistant: Amy Pfund
Composition: S4Carlisle Publishing Services
Printer/Binder: Edwards Brothers Malloy
Cover Printer: Edwards Brothers Malloy
Cover Image: Pete Saloutos/Corbis

CO Credits: 1. Schmid Christophe/Shutterstock; **2.** Monkey Business Images/Shutterstock; **3.** Dmitriy Shironosov/Shutterstock; **4.** Supri Suharjoto/Shutterstock; **5.** moodboard/Alamy; **6.** Monkey Business Images/Shutterstock; **7.** KidStock/Blend Images/Corbis; **8.** Andresr/Shutterstock; **9.** Sergey Rusakov/Shutterstock; **10.** fotosearch/SuperStock; **11.** Sandro Donda/Shutterstock; **12.** Aurora Open/SuperStock; **13.** Gallo Images/SuperStock; **14.** OJO Images/SuperStock; **15.** Fotosearch/Getty Images; **16.** moodboard/SuperStock; **17.** heshphoto/Getty Images; **18.** Exactostock/SuperStock; **19.** Suzanne Tucker/Shutterstock; **20.** Datacraft Co. Ltd/Getty Images; **21.** eurobanks/Shutterstock; **22.** DreamPictures/Shannon Faulk/SuperStock; **23.** KidStock/Blend Images/Getty Images; **24.** heKtor/Shutterstock; **25.** holbox/Shutterstock; **26.** Daniel Goodings/Shutterstock; **27.** Blend Images/SuperStock; **28.** Monkey Business Images/Shutterstock; **29.** Kapu/Shutterstock.

10 9 8 7 6 5 4 3 2 1

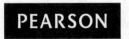

ISBN 10:　　0-13-4070267
ISBN 13: 978-0-13-4070261

Preface

The nursing profession evolves to meet the needs of clients in a continuously changing healthcare environment. The nurse must acquire knowledge and skills and use all available resources and evidence to meet client needs. The nursing process has always guided nurses to practice in an organized and competent manner. Assessment is the first part of this process, and it is the foundation for nursing practice. This *Applications Manual* is designed to accompany the *Health & Physical Assessment in Nursing* (3rd edition) textbook by Donita D'Amico and Colleen Barbarito. It provides the student with opportunities to review the content in the text, reinforce what has been learned, and apply the new knowledge to clinical scenarios and various activities that support critical thinking. It furthers the development of knowledge and skills required when applying the nursing process in clinical practice. The workbook is designed to be used independently, with a laboratory partner, in class, or in study groups. The exercises allow the student to fully engage in each experience.

In each chapter you will find:

- A variety of exercises to reinforce key concepts of the chapter
- Critical thinking exercises that will continuously build on what was learned in previous chapters
- NCLEX®-style review questions

The assessment chapters also include:

- Anatomy and physiology review
- Health history and focused interview exercises
- Scenarios for various age levels that put emphasis on interpretation of findings as normal and abnormal
- Documentation worksheets
- Case studies

The Answer Key for this *Applications Manual* is posted for easy access on the student resources space for *Health & Physical Assessment in Nursing* (3rd edition). By posting the answers online rather than including them within this book, we hope to encourage you to critically think through the exercises before checking your progress. Some of the questions are factual and can be verified in the textbook; others require decision making or application of critical thinking skills. You can locate the downloadable Answer Key at www.pearsonhighered.com/nursingresources.

When a student leaves the classroom or lab, he or she should feel confident that this workbook is a resource that can be used to continue the practice of health assessment skills and to evaluate his or her own progress. Recognizing one's own strengths and weaknesses can be a motivating force for students to push themselves to the next level. We personally challenge each student to be a better nurse than they ever imagined they could be.

Remember the Native American saying that inspired the creation of this workbook: *"Tell me, and I'll forget. Show me, and I may not remember. Involve me, and I'll understand."*

Contents

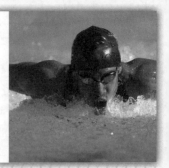

1 Health Assessment

A journey of a thousand miles must begin with a single step.
—Lao Tzu

This chapter addresses introductory concepts for health assessment. The exercises are intended to assist learning and may be assigned for completion by the individual, or as part of classroom activities.

OBJECTIVES

At the completion of these exercises, you will be able to:

1. Define key terminology regarding key anatomic positions.
2. Develop a personal definition of health.
3. Formulate methods to operationalize topic areas of *Healthy People 2020*.
4. Differentiate between and among the various components of the health history.
5. Identify problems with confidentiality in simulated situations.
6. Utilize various documentation methods.
7. Apply critical thinking in analysis of case studies.
8. Differentiate between and among the various roles of the professional nurse.
9. Apply principles of teaching and learning.
10. Complete NCLEX®-style review questions related to the health assessment.

ANATOMIC PLANES TERMINOLOGY

Terminology in Relation to Anatomic Planes

_____ 1. Anterior (ventral)
_____ 2. Cephalad
_____ 3. Distal
_____ 4. Deep
_____ 5. External
_____ 6. Medial
_____ 7. Superior
_____ 8. Supine
_____ 9. Posterior (dorsal)
_____ 10. Caudad
_____ 11. Proximal
_____ 12. Superficial
_____ 13. Internal
_____ 14. Lateral
_____ 15. Inferior
_____ 16. Prone

A. closest to the center or a medial line
B. farther from the midline; toward or on the side
C. below the surface
D. toward the head
E. on or above the surface
F. inside of
G. toward the feet
H. face down
I. outside of
J. toward the front
K. farthest from the center, or a medial line
L. closer to the midline
M. toward the back
N. upper
O. face up
P. lower

DEFINING HEALTH

1. After reviewing the various definitions of health in the textbook, write your own definition of health.

HEALTHY PEOPLE 2020

Healthy People 2020 focuses on improving the health of people living in the United States of America.

1. Using an electronic database, find a current article that relates to any one of the *Healthy People 2020* topic areas.

   Name the news or web source: _____

   Identify the selected focus area: _____

2. Log on to a healthcare agency website (e.g., a local hospital or your local health department). Does the agency offer any programs that relate to or support *Healthy People 2020*'s topic areas? Identify:

   Name the agency: _____

   Name the program: _____

   Explain how the program supports *Healthy People 2020*:

   _____

   _____

3. Consider the students who attend your college or university. Name at least five health issues that affect college students on your campus.

   1.

   2.

   3.

   4.

   5.

4. Identify your top three health concerns on campus.

   1.

   2.

   3.

Program Development

1. Using your list of health concerns from the previous page, describe a program that you would develop to improve the health of your campus community.

2. Present your idea to your class, and ask your peers if they would participate in your proposed program if it were actually offered. What are the rationales for their decisions?

3. Did more than 50% of your class choose to participate? If not, why not?

HEALTH ASSESSMENT

Health History

Match each piece of assessment data in Column A with the appropriate health history component in Column B.

<u>Column A</u>

_____ 1. Father died of cancer

_____ 2. "I'm as strong as an ox"

_____ 3. Denies bloating

_____ 4. Widowed for 10 years

_____ 5. Walks 3 miles, three times per week

_____ 6. Hypertension for 2 years

_____ 7. Felt a pop in the left knee when playing tennis today

_____ 8. Allergic to sulfa-based medications

_____ 9. Smokes 1 ppd (pack per day) × 3 yr

_____ 10. Last BM (bowel movement) 2 days ago

<u>Column B</u>

A. biographical data
B. perceptions about health
C. past history of illness and injury
D. present history of illness and injury
E. family history
F. review of systems
G. health practices

Data

For each piece of data collected, determine the following: Is it subjective or objective? Is it collected during the health history or the physical assessment? Write the appropriate letters on the lines provided to label each piece of information.

S = Subjective   **O** = Objective   **HH** = Health history   **PA** = Physical assessment

1. _____ & _____ Blood pressure 136/80 mmHg in an adult

2. _____ & _____ Client states "I had a fever last night"

3. _____ & _____ Abdomen is soft and nondistended

4. _____ & _____ Lung sounds are clear

5. _____ & _____ Client states "I have so much pain in my right knee"

6. _____ & _____ Client's mother had breast cancer

7. _____ & _____ Heart rate 72 beats per minute (bpm)

8. _____ & _____ Weight 175 lb

9. _____ & _____ Client states "I think I vomited three times last night"

10. _____ & _____ Saliva present in oral cavity

Confidentiality

Put a check next to each scenario where a breach in confidentiality has occurred. Identify the actual breach on the line provided.

_____   1. A nurse is discussing her client's status with a nurse from another unit during lunch in the cafeteria.

Breach _____

_____   2. A nurse is discussing his client's status with an advanced practice nurse in order to improve wound care.

Breach _____

_____   3. A nurse leaves a client's chart open on the desk at the nurses' station while he goes to medicate the client for pain.

Breach _____

_____   4. A nurse looks in the hospital computer system to see if her neighbor has delivered her baby.

Breach _____

_____   5. A nurse pulls up a computerized chart to see why his old girlfriend was admitted through the emergency department.

Breach _____

_____   6. A nurse uses a computerized documentation system and leaves the screen open to a client's medication administration record while she goes to answer a call light.

Breach _____

_____   7. A nurse is contacting the state services for suspected child abuse.

Breach _____

_____   8. A nurse is contacting the sharing network (an organ donation network) about a client who expired.

Breach _____

_____   9. The client in Room 201A asks the nurse about the health condition of his roommate in Room 201B. The nurse explains to him that the roommate is no longer contagious from an infection he had 2 weeks ago.

Breach _____

_____   10. A mother calls the hospital looking for her 23-year-old daughter. The nurse explains to the mother that she was discharged 2 hours ago with her boyfriend.

Breach _____

Documentation

Write the term represented by each standard abbreviation listed.

Example: RUQ = right upper quadrant

1.	Dx	= _____	7.	abd	= _____
2.	Hx	= _____	8.	LMP	= _____
3.	Wt	= _____	9.	CVA	= _____
4.	ADL	= _____	10.	VS	= _____
5.	BP	= _____	11.	WBC	= _____
6.	CBC	= _____	12.	CNS	= _____

Charting

Read the following scenario and document the findings and events using the stated documentation methods.

On a hot summer day Sister Mary Katherine (a 63-year-old female) presents to the emergency department with weakness and a rapid heartbeat. She states she was gardening all day in the church courtyard and never took a break to eat or drink. Her blood pressure (BP) is 86/40 mmHg and her heart rate (HR) is 119 beats per minute (bpm). Her mucous membranes are dry and she cannot recall the last time she urinated. You begin to infuse intravenous fluids as ordered by the healthcare provider. After

2 hours she has received 1 liter of fluid. Her BP is now 109/62 mmHg and her HR is 88 bpm. She was also able to provide a urine sample of 475 ml (clear amber) during this time, which was sent to the lab for a urinalysis test.

1. Using the APIE method of documentation, sort out the information provided to chart the events.

    A

    P

    I

    E

2. Using the same scenario, try to document the events using the SOAP method.

    S

    O

    A

    P

3. Read the following narrative note for this scenario.

    IV fluids were started on client because she showed signs of dehydration. Pt improved upon completion of infusion. Vital signs are stable.

    Is this nurse's note written correctly? If yes, provide rationale. If not, write the note correctly.

THE NURSING PROCESS AND CRITICAL THINKING

In the following scenario, identify information that corresponds to steps in the nursing process.

1. Percy Chan, RN, is a staff nurse on a busy medical-surgical unit. Her client is a 25-year-old female who has had her uterus removed (hysterectomy). The client complains of intermittent sharp pains in the lower abdomen rated as an 8 on a scale of 0–10. After careful questioning, Nurse Chan interprets her findings as "pain related to the surgical incision" and plans to administer 4 mg of morphine to the client. After administering the medication via subcutaneous injection, she returns in 30 minutes to reassess her client's pain status. The client states her pain has decreased and rates it a 2 on a scale of 0–10.

    Assessment

    Diagnosis

    Planning

    Implementation

    Evaluation

Read the scenario below and answer the questions that follow in the space provided.

2. Sally Johnson is a 21-year-old female who has been treated for depression as an outpatient at her county's mental health clinic. She has been taking an antidepressant medication for 6 weeks and has come to the clinic today for a follow-up visit. During the assessment, Sally states she has been feeling more energetic and has more of an appetite than she did on her first visit. However, she has been experiencing dry mouth and frequent headaches.

   A. As the nurse assessing Sally, determine which findings are normal and which findings are abnormal.

   B. Develop a nursing diagnosis based on your findings.

   C. Explain the difference between planning and implementation.

CRITICAL THINKING

Elements of Critical Thinking

Place the following essential elements of critical thinking in the correct order (1 being the first step and 5 being the last).

_____   Selection of alternatives

_____   Analysis of the situation

_____   Collection of information

_____   Evaluation

_____   Generation of alternatives

Application of the Critical Thinking Process

Read the following scenario and answer the questions as you go along.

You are in a gourmet chocolate shop at the mall when you suddenly hear shouts for help and see a crowd of people forming at the entranceway to the shop. You run over to find a young woman on the ground who appears to be unconscious. As a student nurse who is certified in basic life support, you offer to help. A bystander tells you that someone has already called emergency medical services (EMS).

THE CRITICAL THINKING PROCESS BEGINS

Collection of Information

1. What information do you need to collect? (Identify the information as subjective or objective.)

2. How will you obtain this information?

You gather the following information:

The woman is Caucasian and approximately 25 years old. She was shopping with a friend. The friend tells you that the woman has no medical history but is severely allergic to peanuts. Last, she noted her friend was sampling chocolates the store provided. After completing the airway, breathing, and circulation assessment, you find the woman is not breathing and has no pulse.

Analysis of the Situation

1. What normal and abnormal data have you collected?

2. Cluster the data that you have collected and identify any patterns that are forming.

3. List any information that is missing.

4. What are your conclusions?

As you quickly determine that her cardiopulmonary assessment is alarmingly abnormal, you begin the process for cardiopulmonary resuscitation (CPR). However, you then find out important missing information. Another bystander informs you that the woman never ate any chocolate because she witnessed the woman trip and hit her head on a metal display and then fall to the ground, hitting her head again. Are your conclusions starting to change based on the additional data collected?

Generation of Alternatives

1. What are your priorities for this woman?

2. Are there any alternate options for her current treatment?

You decide that your priority remains maintaining her airway, breathing, and circulation. You feel you are tiring and may not be providing CPR as well as you were when you started. You quickly ask if anyone else is capable of performing two-rescuer CPR with you. Another bystander assists you.

Selection of Alternatives

1. What is your continued plan of care?

2. What are your expected outcomes?

Your plan of care is to continue two-rescuer CPR until EMS arrives. At that point you will communicate to the EMS team the information that you have already collected. Your anticipated outcome is that the CPR that has been provided to the woman allowed for adequate oxygenation and circulation in order for her to survive the incident with minimal or no deficits.

Evaluation

1. How can you evaluate the outcome of this scenario?

2. Would you change any of the steps you followed?

> *It may be difficult for you to truly evaluate if the expected outcome will be achieved in this particular kind of scenario given the current environment. The next day it is printed in the newspaper how a shopper saved a woman's life in the mall.*

ROLE OF THE PROFESSIONAL NURSE IN HEALTH ASSESSMENT

Match the role in Column B with the task in Column A. A role may be used more than once.

Column A

_____ 1. Planning a budget to accommodate Medicare reimbursement cutbacks

_____ 2. Orienting staff to new equipment and technology

_____ 3. Conducting a study on the relationship between postpartum depression and spirituality

_____ 4. Educating a community about community-acquired methicillin-resistant *Staphylococcus aureus* (MRSA)

_____ 5. Monitoring the urine output of a postoperative client

_____ 6. Gathering data to prevent ventilator-acquired pneumonia

_____ 7. Repositioning a client in bed to prevent skin breakdown

_____ 8. Reviewing wound care products from vendors to determine which would be the best for the hospital to purchase

Column B

A. nurse caregiver
B. clinical nurse specialist
C. nurse researcher
D. nurse administrator
E. nurse educator

TEACHING PLANS

Objectives

Read each objective. Determine the domain of the objective and circle the appropriate letter.
C = Cognitive   **A** = Affective   **P** = Psychomotor

1. At the completion of this learning session, the student will be able to differentiate among isotonic, hypertonic, and hypotonic solutions.

   C   A   P

2. At the completion of this learning session, the client will be able to demonstrate safe crutch walking.

   C   A   P

3. At the completion of this learning session, the client will be able to avoid foods high in cholesterol.

   C   A   P

4. At the completion of this learning session, the student will be able to calibrate the glucometer.

        C   A   P

5. At the completion of this learning session, the client will be able to assume responsibility for his alcohol consumption.

        C   A   P

6. At the completion of this learning session, the client will be able to name five foods high in *trans* fats.

        C   A   P

7. At the completion of this learning session, the client will be able to state the risk factors for stroke.

        C   A   P

8. At the completion of this learning session, the student will be able to differentiate among the three domains of educational objectives.

        C   A   P

Teaching Methods

Read each learning need and circle the best teaching method to present the content.

1. A community needs to learn about protective measures against West Nile virus:
    Role play   OR   *Lecture*

2. A client needs to learn how to apply a smoking cessation patch:
    Demonstration   OR   *Case study*

3. A mother needs to learn how to breastfeed her baby:
    Practice   OR   *Lecture*

4. A husband needs to learn how to change a dressing on his wife's foot:
    Audiovisual presentation   OR   *Demonstration*

5. A client needs to learn what to expect when she goes in for a nuclear stress test:
    Group discussion   OR   *Printed material*

6. A mother's group needs to learn about stress management techniques after delivering twins:
    Group discussion   OR   *Lecture*

7. A mother needs to learn how to suction her son's tracheostomy at home:
    Role play   OR   *Demonstration*

8. A client needs to learn about the side effects of her chemotherapy:
    Explanation   OR   *Practice*

Teaching Scenario

Read the scenario below and answer the questions that follow in the space provided.

You have been caring for a client with an exacerbation of asthma for 3 days. The client admits to smoking two packs of cigarettes per day for 35 years. You have identified a learning need for this client to stop smoking.

1. Develop a short-term and long-term goal. Explain your response.

2. State the goal(s) for this client.

3. Write one objective from each of the three domains to support one of the goals.

    a.

    b.

    c.

4. Name three specific resources you would use to seek out information when formulating the content for your plan (e.g., scholarly journals, textbooks, websites).

    a.

    b.

    c.

5. One of the teaching methods you have selected is to demonstrate how to apply the nicotine patch. What is the best method to evaluate that learning has taken place? Why?

NCLEX®-STYLE REVIEW QUESTIONS

Read each question carefully. Choose the best answer for each question.

1. The nurse identifies the letters in SOAP charting as:
    1. S—subjective, O—objective, A—analysis, P—prioritizing
    2. S—subjective, O—orders, A—assessment, P—prioritizing
    3. S—signs & symptoms, O—organization of data, A—analysis, P—planning
    4. S—subjective, O—objective, A—assessment, P—planning

2. The nurse understands that charting by exception is a documentation method that is based on: (Select all that apply.)
    1. preestablished norms
    2. the elimination of repetition
    3. the use of phrases and sentences
    4. the frequent use of scales
    5. a computer program

3. The nurse understands the importance of the health history because it:
    1. eliminates the need for a full physical assessment
    2. provides cues and guides for further data collection
    3. saves the nurse time by focusing only on verbal cues
    4. is the basis for formulating the nursing diagnosis

4. The nurse identifies which component(s) in the following statement as variable data?

    A 55-year-old African American male has a blood pressure of 156/80.

    1. Age and BP
    2. Ethnicity and sex
    3. Age and sex
    4. Ethnicity and BP

5. Which of the following activities are the responsibility of the nurse educator? (Select all that apply.)
    1. Teaching a new graduate how to use an IV pump
    2. Coordinating a workshop for critical care nurses
    3. Providing staff nurses with information about a new medication
    4. Writing a grant for funds to conduct research
    5. Assessing the client's daily intake of food

6. The nurse is obtaining a health history from a 67-year-old male with a history of hypertension and diabetes. After obtaining the history of past illness, the next step would be to:
    1. obtain a BP and a fingerstick glucose level
    2. continue with a family history and review of systems
    3. educate the client about a low-sodium, sugar-controlled diet
    4. discuss referring the client to a cardiologist

7. The nurse has developed a teaching plan for a senior center that has requested information on weight-bearing exercises to prevent osteoporosis. The nurse has identified the objectives as being in the psychomotor domain. Which teaching method would be the **least** appropriate choice?
    1. Practice
    2. Demonstration
    3. Case study
    4. Computer-assisted instruction

8. The nurse has completed a comprehensive health assessment on a middle-aged female client. When analyzing the data, the nurse is able to develop clusters. Which cluster has the poorest relationship?
    1. Cough, chest pain, green sputum
    2. Weight loss, poor appetite, "my father passed away 2 weeks ago"
    3. Diarrhea, swelling of the ankles, exercises three times per week
    4. Frequent urination, nocturia, drinks five cups of coffee per day

9. The nurse has just completed a comprehensive health assessment on a 76-year-old female who recently lost her husband of 48 years to stomach cancer 3 months ago. She currently lives alone in the single-family colonial-style home she shared with her husband throughout their marriage. She admits to skipping meals and states, "What's the point of cooking a full meal if I am the only one who will eat it?" She has lost 16 pounds from her already-petite 110-pound frame (height 4′11″). She attends church service every Sunday and has recently started to attend a widows' support group on Thursday evenings. Which behaviors should the nurse interpret as abnormal?
    1. Skipping meals and the widows' support group
    2. Weight loss and living alone
    3. Skipping meals and weight loss
    4. Church services and widows' support group

10. A male client arrives at a preadmission testing center for laboratory work and a chest x-ray 5 days prior to his scheduled back surgery (lumbar laminectomy). He tells the nurse that he is very anxious about his upcoming surgery. The nurse's next step would be to:
    1. take the client on a tour of the perioperative area
    2. ask the client if he has ever had surgery before
    3. instruct the client to obtain a prescription for antianxiety medication
    4. tell the client that he has a great surgeon and has nothing to worry about

2 ▸ Human Development Across the Life Span

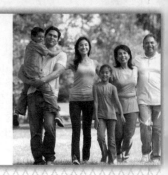

. . . focus on the journey, not the destination. Joy is found not in finishing an activity but in doing it.

—Greg Anderson

This chapter addresses ways in which a variety of factors related to growth and development influence an individual's health. It provides a foundation for assessment and planning nursing interventions appropriate for the age and developmental level of the client.

OBJECTIVES

At the completion of these exercises, you will be able to:

1. Identify assessment findings that are consistent with growth and development milestones.
2. Categorize developmental tasks for various stages of development.
3. Differentiate among the stages of psychosocial theory.
4. Interpret health assessment findings according to growth and development principles.
5. Apply the critical thinking process to case studies.
6. Complete NCLEX®-style review questions related to health assessment across the life span.

DEVELOPMENT MILESTONES

Circle the average age at which a child is expected to achieve each development milestone.

1. Pulls self to standing position

   5 months   8 months   12 months

2. Goes up and down stairs alternating feet

   12 months   2 years   3 years

3. Smiles socially

   2 weeks   2 months   5 months

4. Places objects in mouth

   1 ½ months   3 ½ months   5 ½ months

5. Babbles and coos

   Birth   2 months   4 months

6. Walks alone

   9 months   12 months   18 months

7. Prints name

   1 year   3 years   5 years

8. Plays "peekaboo" and "pat-a-cake"

   4 months   10 months   18 months

9. Says one word

   11 months   18 months   22 months

10. Transfers objects from one hand to another

    3 months   6 months   10 months

11. Sits without support

    5 months   7 months   11 months

12. Cruises

    5 months   10 months   18 months

STAGES OF DEVELOPMENT

Read each developmental task and place the letter representing the appropriate stage of development on each line.

I = Infancy   P = Preschool age   A = Adolescents   M = Middle age

T = Toddler   S = School age   Y = Young adults   O = Older adults

_____ 1. Controlling body functions

_____ 2. Conducting a life review

_____ 3. Coping with children leaving home

_____ 4. Developing a meaningful philosophy of life

_____ 5. Developing hobbies and leisure activities

_____ 6. Preparing for death

_____ 7. Mastering physical skills

_____ 8. Developing a conscience

_____ 9. Differentiating self from others

_____ 10. Interacting with the environment

_____ 11. Forming close relationships with primary caregivers

_____ 12. Developing logical reasoning

_____ 13. Identifying sex role

_____ 14. Searching for identity

_____ 15. Tolerating separation from primary caregivers

_____ 16. Learning to use language for social interaction

_____ 17. Fitting into a peer group

_____ 18. Forming a value system

_____ 19. Beginning a parenting role

_____ 20. Adjusting to aging parents

PSYCHOSOCIAL THEORY

Read each scenario. Write the crisis each person is facing in the space provided. Circle whether or not the nurse would need to intervene. Provide a rationale for your decision.

Crisis Bank

Trust vs. mistrust   Autonomy vs. shame and doubt

Initiative vs. guilt   Industry vs. inferiority

Identity vs. role diffusion   Intimacy vs. isolation

Generativity vs. stagnation   Integrity vs. despair

1. A 5-month-old girl cries when a neighbor holds her, yet coos when returned to her mother's arms.

   Crisis: _____

   Intervention required: Yes or No

   Rationale: _____

2. An 85-year-old man lost his wife of 65 years to cancer 3 months ago. Since her death, he has not attended his Elk's Club meetings and has lost interest in chatting in the evening with his neighbors.

   Crisis: _____

   Intervention required: Yes or No

   Rationale: _____

3. A 35-year-old female is celebrating her 10th wedding anniversary. She is planning a surprise romantic weekend for her husband.

   Crisis: _____

   Intervention required: Yes or No

   Rationale: _____

4. A 55-year-old female has sent her last child off to college. With the free time she will now have, she has decided to start an environmental group in her community to encourage people to "Go Green."

   Crisis: _____

   Intervention required: Yes or No

   Rationale: _____

5. A 4-year-old boy wants to help his father paint the garage. He puts on his overalls, grabs a paintbrush, and exclaims "I'm just like Daddy."

   Crisis: _____

   Intervention required: Yes or No

   Rationale: _____

6. An 18-month-old girl wants to feed and dress herself.

   Crisis: _____

   Intervention required: Yes or No

   Rationale: _____

7. A 17-year-old has decided to apply to college after high school graduation and pursue a career in trauma nursing.

   Crisis: _____

   Intervention required: Yes or No

   Rationale: _____

8. An 8-year-old boy wants to quit the soccer team after attending only four practices. He states "I'll never be any good at sports."

   Crisis: _____

   Intervention required: Yes or No

   Rationale: _____

ASSESSMENT FINDINGS

Items 1 through 10 include health assessment data collected for various age groups. Identify each as normal or abnormal by circling the correct response.

1. Weight at birth is 7.2 lb on July 26; weighs 6.8 lb on July 28.
   Normal   **OR**   **Abnormal**

2. A 56-year-old is sad because her only child is getting married.
   Normal   **OR**   **Abnormal**

3. Height at birth is 21 inches; 1 year later height is 27 inches.
   Normal   **OR**   **Abnormal**

4. A 9-month-old is unable to sit briefly without support.

   Normal   **OR**   **Abnormal**

5. A 10-month-old imitates sounds.

   Normal   **OR**   **Abnormal**

6. A 2½-year-old wants to touch everything in the examination room.

   Normal   **OR**   **Abnormal**

7. A 4-year-old loves to play dress-up.

   Normal   **OR**   **Abnormal**

8. A 75-year-old writes his living will.

   Normal   **OR**   **Abnormal**

9. An 8-year-old begins to have voice changes.

   Normal   **OR**   **Abnormal**

10. A 15-year-old prefers to spend his weekends with his grandparents instead of his peers.

    Normal   **OR**   **Abnormal**

APPLICATION OF THE CRITICAL THINKING PROCESS

Read the following scenario and answer the questions as you go along.

Janie Perkins is a 68-year-old female who arrives at your clinic for an annual physical. She retired 2 weeks ago from her postal job after 40 years of service. She states, "I want to make sure I enjoy a long and healthy retirement with my husband."

1. According to Erikson's psychosocial theory, Janie is facing which maturational crisis?

2. Write three questions you would ask Janie to assess how she is dealing with the developmental tasks she is facing.

   1.

   2.

   3.

Did you ask questions related to Janie's plans for her retirement? What will she be doing with her free time? How does she feel about entering this stage of her life?

After further questioning, Janie tells you she has signed up as a volunteer for the Women's Auxiliary at the local hospital. She has also joined a health club with an interest in starting yoga or Pilates.

3. Which developmental task does this information relate to?

4. Is this a positive or negative response?

> *Janie is developing post-retirement activities that will help her maintain her self-worth and usefulness. This is a positive response for her developmental tasks.*

From the health history, you learn that Janie is lactose intolerant and has not had her cholesterol checked in 10 years.

5. Why is this information important for Janie at this stage of her life?

> *Women over the age of 65 have a decrease in skeletal mass. The decreased density in the bones can lead to brittle bones that may fracture easily. People with lactose intolerance may not be taking in an adequate amount of calcium, which is needed during this time. Heart disease is the leading cause of death among women of this age group. A cholesterol screening is an important part of the care of this client. The nurse should consider a complete nutritional assessment.*

Continuing the health history, you learn that Janie's 88-year-old father lives with her and her husband. Through the years he has been becoming less and less independent and is requiring more supervision. Janie shares this responsibility with her sister, who lives 5 miles away. She is becoming a bit concerned about this situation because her sister is having a total hip replacement in 3 weeks and will require months of rehabilitation.

6. List two questions you would ask Janie to further assess this situation.

   1.

   2.

7. Imagine that Janie lives in your town. Search websites for resources in your community (local hospital, local health department, etc.) and find two resources that would help Janie with this situation.

   1. Name each website.

   2. Describe each resource or program.

   3. Does each resource/program charge a fee?

NCLEX®-STYLE REVIEW QUESTIONS

Read each question carefully. Choose the best answer for each question.

1. When conducting a physical assessment on a 72-year-old client, the nurse must consider which changes in physiological development?
   1. Increased vital capacity
   2. Increased filling and emptying ability of the heart valves
   3. Increase in peripheral vascular resistance
   4. Increased filtering abilities of the kidneys

2. Which teaching topic would be most appropriate for a nurse to plan for an adolescent?
1. Seat belt safety
2. Prostate screening
3. Importance of influenza vaccinations
4. Adjusting to aging parents

3. The nurse understands that myelinization in the spinal cord is almost complete by _____ year(s) of age.
1. 1
2. 2
3. 3
4. 4

4. The nurse is aware that children of low socioeconomic status:
1. have been found to have higher heights and weights than those in other economic groups
2. are more likely to include fresh fruits, vegetables, and lean meats in their diet
3. may have an impaired ability to meet their nutritional needs
4. are less likely to be exposed to environmental elements that influence physical health and well-being

5. The nurse is aware that an appropriate age to give a child a tricycle for his birthday would be:
1. 15 months
2. 1 year
3. 3 years
4. 5 years

6. Which sentence would be age appropriate for the language development of a 3-year-old?
1. "Mama, Mama."
2. "Juice please."
3. "Can I color now?"
4. "Will we be going to the movies today?"

7. A new mother refuses to offer a pacifier to her newborn baby. The nurse is aware that according to Freud's stages of psychosexual development, this affects the:
1. phallic phase
2. latency phase
3. oral phase
4. anal phase

8. A fifth-grade male student visits the school nurse's office of a large urban elementary school each day complaining of various ailments. The nurse speaks with the student's teacher and learns that his grades have been poor and he does not interact with the other children in his class. The nurse's next action should be to:
1. sit down and speak with the student to obtain more information about his home situation
2. refer the student to the school counselor
3. call the student's parents to discuss his school performance
4. instruct the student to discuss with his parents the possibility of starting antidepressants

9. A 3-year-old child enters the clinic with her mother for her annual physical examination. When attempting to assess her blood pressure, the nurse should:
1. state "Let me take your blood pressure."
2. state "I'm going to assess your blood pressure."
3. state "I will be putting this cuff on your arm, and it will start to give your arm a small squeeze."
4. try to distract the child and then quickly put the cuff on without saying anything.

10. Which clients require further assessment by the nurse? (Select all that apply.)
1. A 43-year-old male who lives in the same home he grew up in as a child with his elderly parents and cannot keep a job
2. A 15-year-old female who is unsure of how many sexual partners she has had
3. A 48-year-old female who has undergone more than 20 cosmetic procedures in the past 5 years and has scheduled a liposuction and abdominoplasty next month
4. A 30-year-old female who is unable to maintain an intimate relationship with anyone for longer than 1 month
5. A 45-year-old female who leaves the business world and goes back to college to pursue a career in education

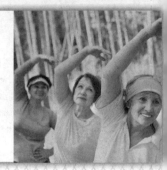

3 Wellness and Health Promotion

It is not the mountain we conquer but ourselves.
—Edmund Hillary

Wellness and health promotion are important areas of focus for today's nurse. Promoting the best possible health is not only cost effective but will increase the quality years of life for our clients and communities. This chapter will assist the student in using theories, models, and frameworks to promote the health of clients, families, and communities.

OBJECTIVES

At the completion of these exercises, you will be able to:

1. Apply wellness theory and health promotion models to client scenarios.
2. Identify immunizations that are appropriate for clients across the life span.
3. Apply critical thinking in analysis of a case study related to wellness and health promotion.
4. Complete NCLEX®-style review questions related to wellness and health promotion.

WELLNESS THEORY

1. Identify the theory represented in the grid provided below _____

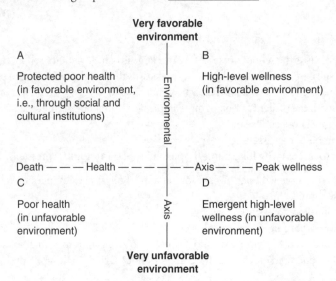

2. Read each of the scenarios below and then apply the above theory to each situation. In the space provided, write the letter (A, B, C, or D) that represents the level of wellness each client is experiencing.

    _____ 1. Victoria is a 45-year-old account executive for a large advertising agency. She has excellent health benefits that include well-visit checkups for general health, vision, and dental health. She runs 3 miles every day after work at her company's fitness center.

_____ **2.** Gerald is a 9-year-old boy with asthma who lives in a homeless shelter with his father. He uses his maintenance inhaler every other day to "make the medicine last" as his father told him to do. He often is seen in the emergency department for upper respiratory infections and has been hospitalized with pneumonia twice in the past the 2 years.

_____ **3.** Kavita is a 22-year-old mother of twin girls (age 15 months). Her husband is currently unemployed and is searching for work. They live in a subsidized housing development in an old urban neighborhood. Kavita walks her daughters in their stroller every day for over an hour. She is using government assistance to make sure she can prepare healthy meals for herself and her family.

_____ **4.** Floyd is a 55-year-old retired semiprofessional baseball player. He lives in an upscale private beach community on the West Coast. He has had a personal trainer for the past 20 years who has kept him physically fit. Recently, Floyd was diagnosed with pancreatic cancer that has metastasized to the bone and brain. He is scheduled to have a feeding tube inserted into his stomach in 2 days.

_____ **5.** Simon is an 81-year-old man who has just auditioned for a reality television show. He lives in an active adult retirement community where he swims daily and likes to participate in various clubs. He has been singing and dancing in his town's holiday pageant every year for the past 10 years.

_____ **6.** Claudia is a 14-year-old girl who has just found out that she is pregnant. She lives in a small two-bedroom apartment with her mother and three other sisters. She smokes marijuana "once in a while" and enjoys drinking alcoholic beverages on the weekends. She is not sure what her plan will be in regard to her pregnancy. She indicates the first step is probably to determine who the father might be.

HEALTH PROMOTION

Read the scenario below and then answer the questions that follow in the space provided.

Richard is a 28-year-old African American who suffers from hypertension. He is obese (weight: 349 lb; height: 5'11"). His mother is obese and has type 2 diabetes. His father died 5 years ago at the age of 52 from complications of diabetes. As a child, Richard did not participate in sports or outdoor activities; rather, he enjoyed his computer and video games. Richard works 10-hour days as an information technology consultant for a software company. His job is very sedentary, and he enjoys going outside for frequent smoke breaks. He has smoked 1.5 packs of cigarettes per day since he was 19. He lives alone and often grabs quick meals at his company's coffee shop or orders take-out meals. Whenever anyone suggests that Richard lose some weight, he replies, "I was born a big boy and I will die a big boy. It's in my genes." Richard did lose 25 lb once when a group of colleagues in his department ran a weight loss contest. With the support of his peers, he found the willpower. Soon after the contest, he regained all of the weight. His company has a fitness center that he does not use. Richard states he is too embarrassed to exercise in the center because his colleagues have made remarks like "Do you think those machines can handle you?" and "Are you trying to fit into your skinny jeans?" Richard also states that it is really hard to lose weight, and he is not really sure how much better his life would be if he did. His mother pushes him to lose weight so he doesn't die young like his father, but this just leads Richard to avoid her.

1. Write your own definition of health promotion.

2. What risk factors for heart disease does Richard have?

3. Which factors can be controlled and which factors cannot? Explain.

4. Use Pender's Health Promotion Model to analyze the information provided in the above scenario. Develop health-promoting behaviors for Richard. Refer to the textbook for model application assistance.

Individual Characteristics and Behaviors	Behavior-Specific Cognitions and Affect	Behavioral Outcome

IMMUNIZATIONS

Circle the immunization that the nurse might prepare for each client who enters the clinic. Draw an X over any immunization that would absolutely NOT be considered for this client.

1. 4-month-old female (no medical history)

   Hep A   **Hib**   **MCV**

2. 15-month-old male (history of gastroesophageal reflux)

   PCV   **DTaP**   **Zoster**

3. 4-year-old male (no medical history)

   Hep B   **RV**   **MMR**

4. 8-year-old female (history of fractured humerus)

   DTaP   **Influenza**   **HPV**

5. 15-year-old female (history of chicken pox—age 4)

   IPV   **Hep B booster**   **HPV**

6. 22-year-old female (4 months pregnant)

   Influenza   **Varicella**   **Zoster**

7. 42-year-old male (history of asthma)

   HPV   **RV**   **Pneumococcal**

8. 60-year-old female (history of HIV)

   Influenza   **IPV**   **MMR**

APPLICATION OF THE CRITICAL THINKING PROCESS

Read the scenario below and then answer the questions that follow in the space provided.

Congratulations, the SmithVille Township Board of Education has just offered you a position as a school nurse in the local high school (grades 9–12). SmithVille Township is a rural area. There are 350 students enrolled in your school for the new academic year.

1. List two primary prevention strategies appropriate for this age group.

   1.

   2.

2. List two secondary prevention strategies appropriate for this age group.

   1.

   2.

To explore the needs of the student body, you decide to have students fill out questionnaires during the first week of school. After analyzing the data, you note the following:

- 35% of the students are sexually active.
- 20% of the students who are sexually active report not using a method of birth control.
- 58% of the students report experimentation with recreational drugs or alcohol.
- 18% of the students report smoking more than one cigarette per day.
- 82% of the students receive fewer than the recommended hours of sleep per night.
- 38% of the students report experiencing anxiety or depression in the past 12 months.
- 5% of the students report having thought about suicide in the past 12 months.

3. Identify a *Healthy People 2020* topic and objective for two of the questionnaire findings.

   1. Finding:

     Topic:

     Objective:

   2. Finding:

     Topic:

     Objective:

4. Discuss your role as the school nurse. Identify two interventions you could implement to promote the health of your students in relation to your selected objectives.

   1.

   2.

5. What other disciplines or organizations would you collaborate with in order to promote the health of these students? Explain.

6. Discuss any barriers you may face (social, financial, administrative, parental, developmental, etc.).

NCLEX®-STYLE REVIEW QUESTIONS

Read each question carefully. Choose the best answer for each question.

1. The nurse defines early identification of illness or disease as:
   1. primary prevention
   2. secondary prevention
   3. tertiary prevention
   4. health promotion

2. The nurse understands tertiary prevention is related to:
   1. prepathology
   2. pathology
   3. rehabilitation
   4. screenings

3. A young adult new mother states, "I just don't think I will be able to breastfeed. It is very complicated and I don't know that I can do it." The nurse interprets this statement as:
   1. low self-efficacy
   2. high self-efficacy
   3. situational influences
   4. interpersonal influences

4. An adult client decides to lose 25 lb. She states, "I joined a gym and signed up at a weight loss center." The nurse can interpret this as:
   1. a commitment without a strategy
   2. a commitment with a strategy
   3. competing demands
   4. behavior-specific cognition

5. A middle-aged adult client smokes two packs of cigarettes per day. When the nurse mentions the health benefits of quitting, the client responds "My mother never smoked a cigarette in her life and died of lung cancer at the age of 48, so what difference does it make?" The nurse interprets this as:
   1. the client is influenced by mother's decision not to smoke
   2. the health promotion behavior should focus on the client's coping with the loss of a parent
   3. the client is experiencing competing demands
   4. the client is unable to perceive a benefit to a health-promoting action

6. The nurse understands that *Healthy People 2020* is a report by:
   1. the Office of Medicare and Medicaid
   2. the Centers for Disease Control and Prevention
   3. the U.S. Department of Health and Human Services
   4. the Joint Commission

7. The nurse is explaining different types of exercise to a group of middle-age adults. The nurse uses the term _____ to describe exercise that includes short periods of vigorous activity.
   1. aerobic
   2. anaerobic
   3. metabolic equivalent
   4. isometric

8. What topic would the nurse be assessing if using the CAGE questionnaire?
   1. Mental health
   2. Substance abuse
   3. Sexual behavior
   4. Injury and violence

9. A young teenager goes to bed at 11:30 p.m. and awakens at 6:30 a.m. for school. The nurse determines that this amount of sleep is:
   1. adequate for his age
   2. inadequate for his age
   3. adequate if a 30-minute nap is included
   4. adequate if a 60-minute nap is included

10. A new mother brings her recently adopted 3-week-old infant to the healthcare provider's office for a well visit. The nurse anticipates that the baby has received which of the following immunizations at birth?
    1. Hib and Hep A
    2. Hep A only
    3. Hep B only
    4. RV and Hep B

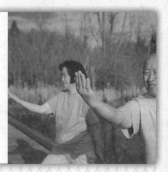

4 Cultural Considerations

What we need to do is learn to respect and embrace our differences until our differences don't make a difference in how we are treated.
—Yolanda King

The United States is historically known as a "melting pot," a multicultural mix of people living together as one society. Nurses are the largest group of healthcare professionals in the United States and have the most direct and continuous contact with clients of all ethnic and cultural backgrounds. Nurses must include attention to the values, beliefs, and customs of clients from diverse cultures in order to plan, provide, and evaluate individualized care. This chapter will review the basic phenomena related to cultural care. It will also help you to develop and utilize a cultural assessment tool.

OBJECTIVES

At the completion of these exercises, you will be able to:

1. Explain the ways in which culture can impact nursing care.
2. Develop a cultural assessment tool.
3. Perform a cultural assessment.
4. Complete NCLEX®-style review questions related to the cultural assessment.

APPLICATION OF THE CRITICAL THINKING PROCESS

Read each of the scenarios below and then answer the questions that follow in the space provided.

Nana Gaya is a 67-year-old African male from Kenya, Africa, who moved to the United States 15 years ago after his daughter married an American soldier from North Carolina. He is fluent in Swahili and is able to speak English very well.

1. List five questions you would ask Mr. Gaya during a cultural assessment.

   1.

   2.

   3.

   4.

   5.

Rachelle is an RN taking care of a 37-year-old female who has large uterine fibroids. The client had heavy vaginal bleeding for over a week before she sought medical attention. Lab values reveal a hemoglobin (Hgb) of 6.2 g/dl and a hematocrit (Hct) of 19.8%. The doctor ordered 2 units of packed red blood cells to be transfused. The client states she is a Jehovah Witness and refuses the blood transfusions. Rachelle remarks in the hallway, "Well, if she bleeds to death it's her own fault! If I were her I would just take the blood and save everyone the trouble."

2. Rachelle's comment can be labeled as:

3. When a client's cultural beliefs and values differ from one's own personal beliefs and values, it is important for the nurse to:

DEVELOPMENT OF THE CULTURAL ASSESSMENT TOOL

Define each component of a cultural assessment and then review the sample question for each component, as listed in Box 4.4 on page 81 of the text. Use the space provided to write two questions that pertain to each component. Once completed, answer your questions to help you to assess your own cultural beliefs and values.

Ethnicity

Define: _____

   1.

   2.

Communication

Define: _____

   1.

   2.

Space

Define: _____

   1.

   2.

Social Organization

Define: _____

   1.

   2.

Time

Define: _____

   1.

   2.

Environment Control

Define: _____

   1.

   2.

Biological Variations

Define: _____

   1.

   2.

PERFORMING THE CULTURAL ASSESSMENT

On a separate sheet of paper, use the cultural assessment tool you developed in the preceding section to assess the cultural beliefs and values of a classmate from a cultural background that is different from your own. Then answer the following questions using the space provided.

1. Describe the nonverbal communication observed during the assessment.

2. How would the use of nonverbal communication by you or your classmate reflect ethnic, cultural, or other factors that may influence the collection of data, analysis of the data, or client care?

3. Compare and contrast your cultural values and beliefs with those of the classmate you interviewed.

NCLEX®-STYLE REVIEW QUESTIONS

Read each question carefully. Choose the best answer for each question.

1. How can a nurse become culturally competent?
    1. By acquiring knowledge and experience
    2. By taking a course on cultural diversity
    3. By researching his or her own culture
    4. By disregarding a client's culture and treating all clients the same

2. The nurse is aware that material culture refers to what factor(s)?
    1. Nonverbal language
    2. Art and clothing
    3. Social structure
    4. Customs

3. According to the World Health Organization (WHO), since 1980 childhood obesity in the United States has changed in what way?
    1. Decreased
    2. Remained the same
    3. Doubled
    4. Tripled

4. An adult Native American client with obesity is seen in an outpatient clinic. Causative factors that the healthcare team might identify could include which of the following factors? (Select all that apply.)
    1. Cultural dietary habits
    2. Lack of exercise
    3. Psychosocial factors
    4. Poverty
    5. Lack of television and Internet service in the home

5. An older adult client who speaks only Italian was hospitalized 2 days ago with abdominal pain. The client is scheduled to go to the operating room for a small-bowel resection. The surgeon is attempting to have the client sign a consent for surgery. The surgeon does not speak Italian. What should the nurse be aware of in terms of this type of situation?
    1. The surgeon is excellent and the client will be just fine
    2. The client can sign the consent now and ask questions later when her family comes in
    3. The client has the right to a translator to provide her information regarding her care
    4. The client is willing to sign the consent; it is her own fault if she does not understand what she is signing

6. An adult Spanish-speaking client is visiting America from Spain. The client twisted her ankle while running on the beach and is being treated in the emergency department. The client's injury is a minor sprain and she is ready to be discharged home. When the nurse provides the client with discharge instructions, it is important for the nurse to do which of the following?
    1. Have the client's 6-year-old daughter translate the instructions because the daughter is able to speak English
    2. Use another English-speaking client who is waiting to be seen to translate
    3. Provide the client with discharge instructions written in Spanish so there is no need to translate anything
    4. Use a bilingual staff member who has been trained in interpretation for clinical purposes

7. Which of the following statements is true about cultural competence education?
    1. Cultural competency is incorporated into the curriculum in nursing education; therefore, it is unnecessary for healthcare agencies to train employees
    2. The U.S. Department of Health and Human Resources has developed a mandatory course that all nurses must complete in order to renew their nursing licenses
    3. All healthcare delivery agencies must develop structures and procedures to address cross-cultural ethical and legal conflicts in healthcare delivery
    4. Only healthcare delivery agencies that serve communities with a large culturally diverse population are required to provide employee training on cultural competence

8. A 21-year-old Muslim girl, whose family has moved to the United States, has enrolled at a community college near her home. She has received permission from her family not to wear her burqa (face veil) to her classes or when she goes out with friends. The girl is exhibiting what type of behavior?
    1. Cultural diversity
    2. Ethnocentrism
    3. Assimilation
    4. Ethnic adoption

9. An adult Vietnamese woman is escorted to the emergency department by her husband when she experiences vaginal bleeding 9 weeks into her pregnancy. Two emergency healthcare providers are available, a male and a female. The male healthcare provider enters the room, and the client's husband kindly requests that his wife be examined by the female healthcare provider. The nurse understands that this request is most likely due to what factor?
    1. A very jealous husband
    2. A bad experience with the male healthcare provider in the past
    3. Clients from the Vietnamese culture having a preference for healthcare providers of the same sex
    4. The husband believing that the female nurse will be able to care for his wife with more compassion

10. An older adult Filipino American is learning to care for his Foley catheter and leg bag at home. While the nurse is explaining how to change the drainage bag, the nurse notices the client continues to nod his head. The nurse would interpret the client's response is what way?
    1. Reassurance that the client understands what is being taught
    2. The client hears what the nurse is saying, but may not understand
    3. A sign that the client probably has done this before
    4. An abnormal response of the central nervous system

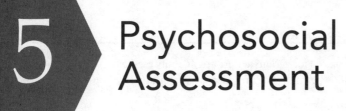

5 Psychosocial Assessment

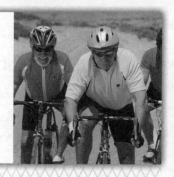

It is confidence in our bodies, mind and spirits that allows us to keep looking for new adventure, new directions to grow in, and new lessons to learn—which is what life is all about.
—Oprah Winfrey

The psychosocial assessment provides the nurse with the information needed to develop an individualized plan of care. It encompasses mental, emotional, social, and spiritual health, which can affect the client's physical well-being. This chapter will allow you to explore factors that can influence psychosocial health and tools that can be used to conduct the assessment.

OBJECTIVES

At the completion of these exercises, you will be able to:

1. Differentiate between internal and external factors that influence psychosocial health.
2. Utilize various psychosocial assessment tools.
3. Interpret psychosocial assessment findings.
4. Develop questions for a psychosocial assessment tool.
5. Complete NCLEX®-style review questions related to the psychosocial assessment.

FACTORS THAT INFLUENCE PSYCHOSOCIAL HEALTH

Identify each piece of data as either an internal factor or external factor to be considered during a psychosocial assessment. Write an "I" for internal or an "E" for external on each line provided.

_____ **1.** Client is living in an urban housing development.

_____ **2.** Client's mother suffers from schizophrenia.

_____ **3.** Client teaches cardio kickboxing 5 days per week.

_____ **4.** Client uses county welfare assistance and has applied for food stamps.

_____ **5.** Client's closest relative lives in Australia.

_____ **6.** Client is living on a farm 50 miles away from the closest hospital.

_____ **7.** Client received a promotion at work and will be receiving a six-figure salary.

_____ **8.** Client's father has alcoholism.

_____ **9.** Client is morbidly obese.

_____ **10.** Client states "I have been under a tremendous amount of stress lately."

_____ **11.** Client smokes two packs of cigarettes per day.

_____ **12.** Client practices yoga and meditation.

_____ **13.** Client has a large extended family involved in her care.

_____ **14.** Client attends a prayer group 3 days per week.

INTERPRETATION OF ASSESSMENT FINDINGS

Items 1 through 10 list psychosocial health assessment data collected for various age groups. Identify each piece of data as normal or abnormal by circling the correct response. Provide a rationale on the line provided for all abnormal findings.

1. A 24-year-old female who states she has had approximately 50 sexual partners

   Normal   or   **Abnormal**

   Rationale: _____

2. A 56-year-old male who looks down to the ground when responding to your questions

   Normal   or   **Abnormal**

   Rationale: _____

3. A 17-year-old female who forces herself to vomit after every meal so she does not gain weight

   Normal   or   **Abnormal**

   Rationale: _____

4. A 30-year-old mother of four who will not take her children to the beach because she admits she does not want to wear a bathing suit in public

   Normal   or   **Abnormal**

   Rationale: _____

5. A 75-year-old male who joins a social group for widows

   Normal   or   **Abnormal**

   Rationale: _____

6. A 45-year-old divorced female who refuses to date because she believes all relationships end in disaster

   Normal   or   **Abnormal**

   Rationale: _____

7. A 48-year-old male who works 80 hours per week and doesn't have much time for his family

   Normal   or   **Abnormal**

   Rationale: _____

8. A 16-year-old male who becomes angry and verbally abusive with others very quickly

   Normal   or   **Abnormal**

   Rationale: _____

9. A 22-year-old female who starts a volunteer group in her neighborhood to provide underprivileged children with recycled sports and dance equipment

   Normal   or   **Abnormal**

   Rationale: _____

10. A 62-year-old female who will not leave the house unless her husband is with her

Normal or **Abnormal**

Rationale: _____

PSYCHOSOCIAL ASSESSMENT TOOLS

Spiritual Assessment

Read each question listed in the HOPE Approach to Spiritual Assessment. In the space provided, write an additional question related to spirituality for each component. When you complete the questions, utilize them to assess the spirituality of your lab partner or a family member.

HOPE APPROACH TO SPIRITUAL ASSESSMENT

H (Spiritual Resources)

1. What are your sources of hope or comfort?
2. What helps you during difficult times?
3. _____

Data collected: _____

O (Organized Religion)

1. Are you a member of an organized religion?
2. What religious practices are important to you?
3. _____

Data collected: _____

P (Personal Spirituality)

1. Do you have spiritual beliefs separate from those of an organized religion?
2. What spiritual practices are most helpful to you?
3. _____

Data collected: _____

E (Effect on Care)

1. Is there any conflict between your beliefs and the care you will be receiving?
2. Do you hold beliefs or follow practices that you believe may affect your care?
3. _____

Data collected: _____

Suicide Assessment

Read the scenario below and then answer the questions that follow in the space provided.

Steven is a 23-year-old Native American who spends most evenings at the local bar. He has recently moved back home with his mother, Sasha. Sasha has suffered from anxiety and depression ever since her husband, Steven's father, committed suicide 5 years ago. Steven is a college graduate who majored in finance. After college he received a great job with a financial planning firm where he worked for 2 years before he was fired 8 months ago. His long-term girlfriend has decided to leave him because she claims he has lost focus and has no direction since he has been laid off. While ordering his fifth beer for the night, he confides to the bartender "What the hell do I have left to live for?"

1. List four characteristics that Steven has that increase his risk for suicide.

   a.

   b.

   c.

   d.

2. Develop three assessment questions the nurse should ask Steven to further explore his risk for suicide.

   a.

   b.

   c.

Stress Assessment

Read the scenario below and then answer the questions that follow in the space provided.

Madison is a 42-year-old female whom you (the nurse) will assist to complete the Holmes Social Readjustment Scale. She reveals the following information: Her husband recently passed away from pancreatic cancer. She is very worried about how she will support her two small children (Isabel, 3 years old, and Harry, 4 months old). Her husband had always supported her, and she has minimal working skills. She can no longer keep up with paying the medical bills and has not paid the mortgage in months. She fears her home will go into foreclosure next month. Her husband's parents have decided to come and stay with her during this difficult time, especially with Christmas approaching. Although their gesture is sincere, Madison does not get along well with her mother-in-law. She has been so busy caring for her children and trying to find work that she has not been able to attend her junior women's club meetings or play tennis with her friends. To make matters worse, she received a ticket and had her car towed for parking in a handicapped parking spot at the supermarket. She has not had a good night's sleep in months.

1. Circle an "Event Value" for each stressor on the Holmes Social Readjustment Scale (provided on page 32) that Madison is experiencing. What is Madison's total score?

   Score: _____

2. List five physical signs that Madison may experience related to her stress level.

   a.

   b.

   c.

   d.

   e.

3. List two questions you would ask Madison to further assess her stress level.

   a.

   b.

4. Imagine that Madison comes to you for help managing her stress. Using available resources (web, community publications, etc.), find a stress management program in your community that she would be able to attend.

   a. Program information:

      i. Title:

      ii. Sponsor:

      iii. Location:

      iv. Cost:

Holmes Social Readjustment Scale

EVENT	EVENT VALUE	
1. Death of a spouse	100	**Directions for completion:** Add up the point values for each of the events that you have experienced during the past 12 months.
2. Divorce	73	
3. Marital separation	65	
4. Jail term	63	**Scoring**
5. Death of a close family member	63	*Below 150 points:*
6. Personal injury or illness	53	The amount of stress you are experiencing as a result of changes in your life is normal and manageable. There is only a 1 in 3 chance that you might develop a serious illness over the next 2 years based on stress alone. Consider practicing a daily relaxation technique to reduce your chance of illness even more.
7. Marriage	50	
8. Fired at work	47	
9. Marital reconciliation	45	
10. Retirement	45	
11. Change in health of family member	44	
12. Pregnancy	40	*150 to 300 points:*
13. Sex difficulties	39	The amount of stress you are experiencing as a result of changes in your life is moderate. Based on stress alone, you have a 50/50 chance of developing a serious illness over the next 2 years. You can reduce these odds by practicing stress management and relaxation techniques on a daily basis.
14. Gain of a new family member	39	
15. Business readjustment	39	
16. Change in financial state	38	
17. Death of a close friend	37	
18. Change to different line of work	36	*Over 300 points:*
19. Change in number of arguments	35	The amount of stress you are experiencing as a result of changes in your life is high. Based on stress alone, your chance of developing a serious illness during the next 2 years approaches 90%, unless you are already practicing good coping skills and regular relaxation techniques. You can reduce the chance of illness by practicing coping strategies and relaxation techniques daily.
20. Mortgage or loan over $10,000	31	
21. Foreclosure of mortgage or loan	30	
22. Change in responsibilities at work	29	
23. Son or daughter leaving home	29	
24. Trouble with in-laws	29	
25. Outstanding personal achievement	28	
26. Spouse begins or stops work	26	
27. Begin or end school	26	
28. Change in living conditions	25	
29. Revision of personal habits	24	
30. Trouble with boss	23	
31. Change in work hours or conditions	20	
32. Change in residence	20	
33. Change in schools	20	
34. Change in recreation	19	
35. Change in church activities	19	
36. Change in social activities	19	
37. Change in sleeping habits	16	
38. Change in number of family get-togethers	15	
39. Vacation	13	
40. Christmas	12	
41. Minor violations of the law	11	
Total Points		

Source: Reprinted from Holmes, T., & Rahe, R. J. (1967). Social Readjustment Rating Scale. *Journal of Psychosomatic Research, 11,* 213–218. Copyright 1967, with permission from Elsevier.

The Psychosocial Assessment

Recall the information in the text regarding the psychosocial assessment. Formulate two of your own questions for each component of the psychosocial assessment. When complete, use the questions to assess the psychosocial health of your lab partner.

Physical Fitness

1.

2.

Data collected: _____

Self-Concept

1.

2.

Data collected: _____

Family History

1.

2.

Data collected: _____

Culture

1.

2.

Data collected: _____

Geography

1.

2.

Data collected: _____

Economic Status

1.

2.

Data collected: _____

Roles and Relationships

1.

2.

Data collected: _____

Stress and Coping

1.

2.

Data collected: _____

Spiritual and Belief Patterns

1.

2.

Data collected: _____

Sort the data collected in your psychosocial assessment of your lab partner by placing it in the categories listed below:

Client Strengths   **Client Weaknesses**

NCLEX®-STYLE REVIEW QUESTIONS

Read each question carefully. Choose the best answer for each question.

1. When a nurse gathers data about the mental, emotional, social, and spiritual well-being of a client, what type of assessment or screening is the nurse performing?
   1. Psychosocial assessment
   2. Psychological screening
   3. Mental health assessment
   4. Cultural assessment

2. The nurse is about to begin an assessment on a female who has been hospitalized for depression. The nurse greets the client by saying "Hello, Mrs. Rodriguez." The client responds by rocking back and forth in her chair while repeating "Hello, hello, hello, hello." The client does not stop until the nurse instructs her to stop. What is this abnormal speech pattern associated with an altered thought process called?
   1. Word salad
   2. Flight of ideas
   3. Circumlocution
   4. Echolalia

3. An adult homeless client has been experiencing frequent chest pain and palpitations. The client has gone to the local emergency department three times in the past month. The client's medical workups have been negative. Which intervention would be most appropriate for this client at this time?
   1. Further assessment of the client's psychosocial status
   2. A prescription for an analgesic due to chest pain
   3. Education on a caffeine-free diet
   4. Education on stroke prevention

4. The nurse recognizes which of the following as physical signs of stress? (Select all that apply.)
   1. Decreased blood clotting time
   2. Dilated bronchi
   3. Elevated blood pressure
   4. Decreased blood supply to vital organs
   5. Constricted pupils

5. The nurse is aware that self-concept is composed of which two components?
   1. Body image and interdependence
   2. Role function and self-esteem
   3. Body image and self-esteem
   4. Role function and interdependence

6. An adult woman has recently lost her only daughter to an aggressive form of brain cancer. Her husband has brought her to the emergency department because he is concerned for her well-being. He states that on multiple occasions he has witnessed his wife talking to the air as if she was talking to their daughter. Which question would be appropriate to help assess if this client is in touch with reality?
   1. "Do you know where you are right now?"
   2. "Do you feel well today?"
   3. "What is your husband's name?"
   4. "Do you miss your daughter?"

7. A 6-year-old boy is frequently in trouble at school. He screams and hits the other children and is very disrespectful to the teachers. The school nurse is concerned about this behavior for what reason? (Select all that apply.)
   1. The child's home environment may influence how he copes with stress at school
   2. The child may have witnessed or may be the victim of some form of abuse in the home
   3. The child obviously does not like his teacher
   4. The child does not know how to make friends
   5. The child is demonstrating a developmental delay

8. After a nurse collects data for a psychosocial assessment, what would be the next step?
   1. Make referrals to community resources
   2. Determine the nursing diagnosis
   3. Sort, group, and categorize the data
   4. Evaluate the plan of care

9. An adult client states, "The voices in my head are telling me to kill people." What is the client experiencing?
   1. Command hallucination
   2. Illusion
   3. Delusion
   4. Somatic hallucination

10. An adult client is a successful financial analyst. She is very attractive and outgoing. She has high self-esteem and is confident that she will achieve her goal of writing a book by the time she is 40. Who is she most likely to seek a relationship with?
    1. A 38-year-old Harvard Law graduate
    2. A 20-year-old who lives at home with his parents while he works on writing a comic book series
    3. An unemployed 54-year-old
    4. A 42-year-old married man with three children

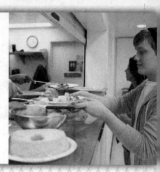

6 Assessment of Vulnerable Populations

Never believe that a few caring people can't change the world. For, indeed that's all who ever have.
—Margaret Mead

Vulnerable populations, living on the fringe of our society, are isolated from many of the basic services that most Americans take for granted. Nurses often work with individuals in these populations in various healthcare settings. Just as cultural considerations of a population must be respected and honored, individuals in vulnerable populations may have needs and beliefs that are outside of the nurse's comfort zone. Awareness of different vulnerable populations will assist the nurse to provide quality care to the individual client.

OBJECTIVES

At the completion of these exercises, you will be able to:

1. Interpret assessment findings of a vulnerable population.
2. Develop questions appropriate for an identified vulnerable population.
3. Identify health disparities related to particular vulnerable populations.
4. Complete NCLEX®-style review questions related to the assessment of vulnerable populations.

FACTS AND FINDINGS

Read each statement below. Recall the descriptions of vulnerable populations in the text. Determine if the statement agrees or disagrees with the text by writing "A" for agrees and "D" for disagrees on each line provided. If the statement does not agree, rewrite it to reflect the text.

_____ 1. Almost all American Indian and Alaska Native people have access to health services through the Indian Health Service.

_____ 2. Coining and cupping are cultural practices that are viewed by healthcare providers as a type of physical abuse.

_____ 3. Elder abuse cannot legally be committed by a family member.

_____ 4. Individuals who identify as lesbian, gay, bisexual, or transgender are at an increased risk of being bullied.

_____ 5. A mixed-status family is a family with one or more family members who are undocumented immigrants and other family members who are citizens, lawful permanent residents, or immigrants with another form of temporary legal immigration status.

_____ 6. The female prison population has been steadily decreasing at a rate faster than that of the male prison population rate.

_____ 7. Two factors that have greatly impacted homelessness during the past 25 years are decreased availability of affordable housing and increased poverty rates.

_____ 8. Caring for individuals from vulnerable populations does not require the nurse to be culturally competent to provide quality nursing care.

_____ 9. Childhood poverty rates have been frozen during the past decade.

_____ 10. Family caregivers caring for aging adults in the home setting have higher rates of depression and anxiety.

APPLICATION OF THE CRITICAL THINKING PROCESS

Read each of the client scenarios below and then answer the questions that follow in the space provided.

1. A young adult female is being seen in the clinic. The nurse notices various stages of bruises on her back, legs, and arms. List five assessment questions that would be appropriate to ask the client in this clinical situation.

   a.

   b.

   c.

   d.

   e.

2. An adult male who is homeless is being seen in the clinic. He has been diagnosed with pneumonia and has a follow-up appointment scheduled for tomorrow. List five concerns the nurse could have regarding the situation.

   a.

   b.

   c.

   d.

   e.

3. Recall the information in your text regarding vulnerable populations. Formulate two of your own general questions for each component noted below.

   a. Race/ethnicity—Native Hawaiian and Other Pacific Islander

      1.

      2.

b. Age—elder abuse

1.

2.

c. Intimate partner violence (IPV)

1.

2.

d. Socioeconomic status—immigrants and refugees

1.

2.

e. Incarcerated men and women

1.

2.

f. Geography—urban/metropolitan area

1.

2.

NCLEX®-STYLE REVIEW QUESTIONS

Read each question carefully. Choose the best answer for each question.

1. Vulnerable populations are not well integrated into the healthcare system because of what factors? (Select all that apply.)
   1. Political views
   2. Ethnicity
   3. Age
   4. Geography
   5. Disabilities

2. Which of the following is **not** a factor of concern in the American Indian and Alaska Native populations?
   1. American Indians have a high infant death rate
   2. The percentage of adults living in poverty is high
   3. Alzheimer's disease is a leading cause of death
   4. American Indians have a high rate of binge drinking

3. A Vietnamese school-age client comes to the clinic, with the mother, with complaints of having a low-grade fever, productive cough, and congestion for 4 days. The nurse pulls up the client's shirt to auscultate the chest and finds long, bilateral scratches across the client's back. What is the nurse's first response?
    1. Do not address the situation, but tell the healthcare provider before the clients enter the room
    2. Ask the mother about the marks on the client's back
    3. Contact social services immediately
    4. Assume the child is being abused, but ask more questions first

4. An elderly client who often visits the clinic by herself arrives today with a nonfamily caregiver whom the nurse has not met before. The caregiver appears to aggressively answer all of the questions directed toward the client. The client's body language is different from previous visits. The client is not looking at the nurse, and her appearance is disheveled, with a strong body odor. Which of the following actions would be a priority for the nurse?
    1. Have the client provide a urine sample to rule out a urinary tract infection
    2. Assess the client for a possible recent stroke
    3. Report the findings to the healthcare provider
    4. Speak with the caregiver and suggest giving the client a bath more often

5. An older adult client is the primary caregiver for a spouse who has dementia. The nurse knows that the client is at risk for which of the factors listed below due to being the primary caregiver? (Select all that apply.)
    1. Depression
    2. Low self-esteem
    3. Anxiety
    4. Social isolation
    5. Weight gain

6. A nurse is working in a women's prison clinic. The nurse knows that women in prison have higher rates of some chronic diseases than the general female population. Which of the following would the nurse expect to see more often in women in prison?
    1. Hepatitis
    2. Lupus
    3. Arthritis
    4. Breast cancer

7. The nurse providing care to a client from a vulnerable population must be aware of what concept to provide quality care?
    1. Cultural competence
    2. Cultural awareness
    3. Cultural heritage
    4. Cultural ethnicity

8. The nurse is aware that psychological abuse can manifest itself in the client in a variety of ways. Which of the following are examples of how abuse can manifest? (Select all that apply.)
    1. Depression
    2. Low self-esteem
    3. Eagerness to please others
    4. Attention-seeking behavior
    5. Withdrawal

9. Which of the following are adolescent behaviors that contribute to death and disability among youths and adults?
    1. Tobacco, alcohol, and other drug use
    2. Involvement in extracurricular activities in school or church
    3. Employment in the fast-food industry
    4. Safe driving habits

10. The nurse is meeting an LGBT client for the first time. How does the nurse greet the client?
    1. Address the client in neutral nongender terminology
    2. Address the client by his or her physical appearance
    3. Address the client by his or her gender assigned by birth
    4. Address the client by how the client identifies he or she wishes to be addressed

Interviewing and Communication Techniques

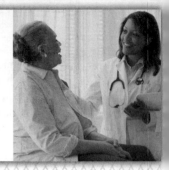

We must know what knowledge is available, how we can obtain it, and why it is true.
—Socrates

By utilizing effective communication skills, the nurse will be able to collect data regarding a client's health status. Demonstrating professionalism throughout all phases of the interview process is vital. This chapter will provide you the opportunity to develop interviewing and communication skills with clients from diverse backgrounds across the entire life span.

OBJECTIVES

At the completion of these exercises, you will be able to:

1. Utilize communication skills.
2. Identify barriers to the communication process.
3. Identify interactional skills used when interviewing and communicating with clients.
4. Differentiate between the phases of the health assessment interview.
5. Identify variations incorporated into the interview process for pediatric and older adult patients.
6. Apply the critical thinking process to case studies and scenario questions.
7. Complete NCLEX®-style review questions related to the interviewing and communication techniques.

INTERACTIONAL SKILLS

Write the definition of each interactional skill on the line provided. Provide an example of each interactional skill.

1. **Attending:** _____

   Example: _____

   _____

2. **Paraphrasing:** _____

   Example: _____

   _____

3. **Direct leading:** _____

   Example: _____

   _____

4. **Focusing:** _____

   Example: _____

   _____

5. **Questioning:** _____

   Example: _____

   _____

6. **Reflecting:** _____

   Example: _____

   _____

7. **Summarizing:** _____

   Example: _____

   _____

BARRIERS TO COMMUNICATION

Read each dialogue and decide whether the nurse was therapeutic or nontherapeutic in his or her response by circling your answer. If the response was nontherapeutic, state the barrier and provide an alternate therapeutic response on the line provided.

1. *Client:* "I am so worried about my upcoming surgery tomorrow morning. I keep thinking something bad is going to happen."

   Nurse: "Don't waste another minute worrying about it. You will be just fine."

   Therapeutic   **Nontherapeutic**

   Barrier: _____

   Alternate Response: _____

   _____

2. *Client:* "I've had pain in my leg for the past few days."

   Nurse: "Do you have any history of peripheral vascular disease (PVD) or venous thromboembolism (VTE)?"

   Therapeutic   **Nontherapeutic**

   Barrier: _____

   Alternate Response: _____

   _____

3. *Client:* "Yesterday my healthcare provider spoke to me so fast when explaining the procedure planned for me tomorrow. I'm a bit concerned."

   Nurse: "It sounds like you may have some questions. Let me see if I can help clarify things for you."

   Therapeutic   **Nontherapeutic**

   Barrier: _____

   Alternate Response: _____

   _____

4. *Client:* "When I started having pain in my chest at 2 a.m., I figured it was just indigestion from the fried food I ate for dinner last night."

   Nurse: "So you also figured you were a doctor last night, too."

   Therapeutic   **Nontherapeutic**

   Barrier: _____

   Alternate Response: _____

   _____

5. *Client:* "I cried all night last night thinking about how my cancer has spread. I'm just not ready to die. I feel like I haven't even truly lived."

   Nurse: "Oh, you should have watched the show I was watching last night on the comedy channel. My husband and I couldn't stop laughing."

   Therapeutic   **Nontherapeutic**

   Barrier: _____

   Alternate Response: _____

   _____

6. *Client:* "My husband was so angry with me last night and totally lost control."

   Nurse: "Let's discuss what you mean by lost control."

   Therapeutic   **Nontherapeutic**

   Barrier: _____

   Alternate Response: _____

7. *Client:* "I think I had sex with someone who has a sexually transmitted disease."

   Nurse: "What makes you think that? Did you use any form of protection? How many partners have you had? Do you have a history of sexually transmitted disease?"

   Therapeutic   **Nontherapeutic**

   Barrier: _____

   Alternate Response: _____

   _____

8. *Client:* "It seems that diabetes is really much more serious than I thought. I'm going to have to rethink a lot of things I do each day."

   Nurse: "It sounds like you have some concerns about your diabetes. Would you like to discuss some of those concerns now?"

   Therapeutic   **Nontherapeutic**

   Barrier: _____

   Alternate Response: _____

   _____

HEALTH HISTORY INTERVIEW: TRUE OR FALSE

Read each statement and decide whether it is true or false. Circle your answer. If the answer is false, rewrite the statement to make it true.

1. The client is the most reliable source of information.

   True   **False**

   Correction: _____

2. Healthcare professionals may be considered secondary sources of information.

   True   **False**

   Correction: _____

3. Pain may affect the client's ability to participate in the interview.

   True   **False**

   Correction: _____

4. It is better to obtain a sexual history early on in the interview to get a potentially embarrassing portion completed first.

   True   **False**

   Correction: _____

5. If a client reports identifying with American culture, further questioning is necessary.

   True   **False**

   Correction: _____

APPLICATION OF THE CRITICAL THINKING PROCESS

Read the scenario below and then answer the questions that follow in the space provided.

Scott Petrowski is a 38-year-old male who has cerebral palsy. He is being admitted to a long-term care facility by his mother, Magda Petrowski, who states she is getting too old to care for him by herself at home. The nurse is preparing to obtain a comprehensive health history as part of the admission process. The nurse is aware that this can be a very stressful time for both mother and son.

1. List three ways the nurse can help reduce the fears and anxiety of the client and family during this time.

   1.

   2.

   3.

2. What sources of data may be used to conduct this interview?

Mrs. Petrowski states multiple times in the interview that she is very upset about having Scott leave her home. She holds his hand throughout much of the interview, and the nurse notes that at times her eyes become very teary.

3. Identify two ways the nurse can show empathy during this interview.

   1.

   2.

The nurse asks questions regarding the client's cultural beliefs, traits, and traditions. Mrs. Petrowski explains they are from a strong Polish family but is confused as to why this is so important for them to know.

4. The nurse responds by stating:

After 1 hour of continuous questioning, it is evident that Scott is becoming very restless. Mrs. Petrowski explains that he usually has his lunch at this time and does not like to stay in his wheelchair for long periods of time. The nurse is aware that the process is only about three-fourths complete.

5. The nurse's best action in this situation would be to:

HEALTH ASSESSMENT INTERVIEW

Name:_____   Date:_____

Age: _____   Gender: _____   Height: _____   Weight: _____

Allergies (medications/food/latex/other): _____

Growth and developmental considerations: _____

Spoken language: _____

Oriented to:

     Person? Y/N

     Place? Y/N

     Date? Y/N

     Purpose? Y/N

Primary source of information: _____

List secondary sources of information: _____

PREINTERACTION

Nurse shift report:

_____

_____

_____

REVIEW OF MEDICAL RECORD:

Past medical history: _____   Surgeries: _____

Reason for today's visit: _____

Medications: _____

Immunizations: _____

General health: _____

Cultural/religious/ psychosocial considerations: _____

INITIAL INTERVIEW

Complete health history form (See Chapter 8, **Health History**)

FOCUSED INTERVIEW

Clarify data as needed.

Describe patient's symptoms in detail using OLDCART & ICE acronyms.

O = Onset _____

L = Location _____

D = Duration _____

C = Characteristics _____

A = Aggravating factors _____

R = Relieving factors _____

T = Treatment _____

&

I = Impact on ADLs _____

C = Coping strategies _____

E = Emotional response _____

LIFESPAN CONSIDERATIONS

Pediatric Patients:

Relationship of patient to adult who presents with child: _____

Pertinent lab data: _____

Older Adult Patients:

Assistive devices? (Specify—glasses, hearing aids, etc.): _____

Patient's preferred title: _____

Pain? (If yes, describe in detail): _____

Other distractions? (Describe—medication side effects, fatigue, anxious, etc.)

_____

Phases of the Health Assessment Interview

Define the purpose of each stage of the health assessment interview.

1. **Phase I—Preinteraction**:

_____

_____

_____

2. **Phase II—The Initial Interview**:

_____

_____

3. **Phase III—The Focused Interview**:

_____

_____

LIFESPAN CONSIDERATIONS

Read the scenario below and then answer the questions that follow in the space provided.

The nurse is preparing for the interview and physical assessment of a 91-year-old patient who is hospitalized for pneumonia. The patient is awake, alert, and oriented and has good long- and short-term recall. The patient's son brought his father to the hospital and remains with him.

1. Is it necessary for the patient's 58-year-old son to be present during the initial interview? Why or why not?

2. What are some ways the nurse can establish rapport and create an optimal environment for the interview and physical assessment?

NCLEX®-STYLE REVIEW QUESTIONS

Read each question carefully. Choose the best answer for each question.

1. A client is injured after falling from a bicycle. The best question for the nurse to include when attempting to gather more details about a client's injuries would be:
   1. "Did you fall on concrete?"
   2. "Do you think you broke any bones?"
   3. "Can you describe how you landed when you fell off the bike?"
   4. "Are you having any pain now?"

2. The nurse understands the term used to select words, body language, and signs to develop a message is called:
   1. encoding
   2. transmitting
   3. decoding
   4. interactional skills

3. A new graduate nurse has just started working in a woman's health clinic where many of the clients speak very little English. The nurse often uses a translator in order to conduct her interviews. When using a translator it is important for the nurse to:
   1. look at the translator while speaking clearly to him or her
   2. pause frequently
   3. speak loudly with more hand gestures than normal
   4. ask the translator to use any slang or idiomatic language

4. A young adult is carried into the emergency department by two friends. The client is barely conscious. The nurse suspects some form of substance abuse. The nurse attempts to obtain information from the client's friends, who are very hesitant to share any information. This is most likely because they:
   1. are a secondary source of information and may not be reliable
   2. have had bad past experiences in the emergency department
   3. fear legal implications
   4. are embarrassed for their friend

5. The nurse identifies which of the following situations as one where a client health history may be impossible to obtain?
   1. A 90-year-old male admitted through the emergency department from a nursing home with no family present
   2. A 6-month-old infant who was left in a safe haven crib at a church
   3. A 36-year-old female who arrives at the hospital in active labor
   4. A 76-year-old female who is in a rehabilitation facility for a stroke she had 3 months ago that has left her with expressive aphasia

6. A 25-year-old female has brought a 4-year-old male to the emergency department complaining of shortness of breath. What is the nurse's priority question?
    1. "Does the child have a history of asthma?"
    2. "What is your relationship to this child?"
    3. "Has he been around other children who are sick?"
    4. "What medications does he take?"

7. The nurse has received the shift report on a client diagnosed with renal failure. The nurse reviews the client's laboratory data and medical history before entering the room. Which phase of the health assessment interview has the nurse completed?
    1. Initial
    2. Focused
    3. Primary
    4. Preinteraction

8. During an interview, a client denies having any medical history. Later, the client states, "I've been taking blood pressure medication for 10 years." The nurse's response should be:
    1. "Tell me the reason your healthcare provider has prescribed blood pressure medication for you."
    2. "What you are saying to me does not make any sense."
    3. "Why are you taking blood pressure medication?"
    4. "You realize that if you are taking blood pressure medication you have a history of high blood pressure, right?"

9. A woman calls the health center stating that there is something wrong with her son's penis. She uses slang terminology during the phone call. The nurse's most professional response would be:
    1. "Ma'am, I will not continue this conversation with you unless you use the proper terminology."
    2. "I would just like to clarify that you are referring to your son's penis."
    3. Hang up the phone; it is most likely a prank call
    4. Use the same terminology with which the client is comfortable

10. The nurse is interviewing a client when the patient suddenly moves back in the chair and crosses her arms and legs. What is the nurse's best action?
    1. Ask the client if she needs to be excused to the bathroom
    2. Move back until the client seems more relaxed
    3. Tell the client the interview will be over in a few minutes
    4. End the interview and begin the physical exam

8 ▶ The Health History

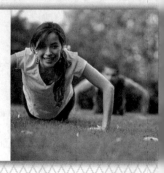

> *We must know what knowledge is available, how we can obtain it, and why it is true.*
> —Socrates

The ability to conduct a comprehensive health history is an important aspect of nursing. Utilizing effective communication skills, the nurse will be able to collect data regarding a client's health status. This chapter will provide you the opportunity to develop communication and documentation skills while learning the components of the health history.

OBJECTIVES

At the completion of these exercises, you will be able to:

1. List the components of the health history.
2. Interpret a pedigree.
3. Develop interview questions for each component of the health history.
4. Complete a focused health history form based on a given scenario.
5. Obtain and document a complete health history.
6. Complete NCLEX®-style review questions related to the health history.

COMPONENTS OF THE HEALTH HISTORY

Write at least one question that may be asked for each component of the health history in the space provided.

1. **Biographical Data**

2. **Present Health or Illness**

3. **Past History**

4. **Family History**

5. **Psychosocial History**

6. **Review of Body Systems**

   Skin

   Hair

   Nails

   Head

   Neck

   Lymphatics

   Eyes

   Ears

   Nose

   Mouth and Throat

   Respiratory

Breasts and Axillae

Cardiovascular

Peripheral Vascular

Abdomen

Urinary

Male Reproductive

Female Reproductive

Musculoskeletal

Neurologic

PEDIGREE

1. Review the pedigree below and answer the following questions. Use the pedigree symbols listed in Chapter 8 of your text.

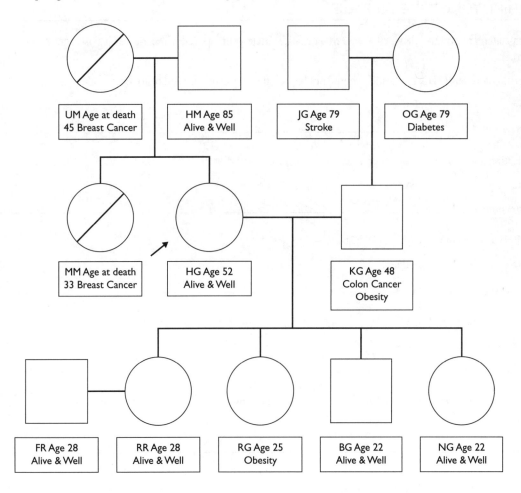

1. What are the initials of the client being interviewed?

2. How many women are in this family?

3. How many generations are represented in this genogram?

4. How many people are deceased in this family?

5. How many siblings does the client have?

6. What disease or illness is this client at risk for?

7. How can this pedigree be used to improve the health of this client?

HEALTH HISTORY: TRUE OR FALSE

Read each statement and decide whether it is true or false. Circle your answer. If the answer is false, rewrite the statement to make it true.

1. Over-the-counter (OTC) medication should not be included in the medication history.

   True   **False**

   Correction: _____

2. Collecting information about a client's health insurance is not part of the health history.

   True   **False**

   Correction: _____

3. Birthplace is part of the psychosocial history.

   True   **False**

   Correction: _____

4. Asking about a client's financial status is inappropriate and unnecessary in healthcare.

   True   **False**

   Correction: _____

5. The client's own words should never be used when documenting any portion of the health history.

   True   **False**

   Correction: _____

DOCUMENTATION SCENARIO

Read the scenario below and then answer the questions that follow in the space provided.

A 24-year-old new mother brings her 2-week-old daughter to the well-baby clinic for a routine visit. The mother received prenatal care, took a prenatal vitamin once per day, and gained 28 lb throughout the pregnancy. She delivered her child by normal vaginal delivery at 38 weeks' gestation. She has been breastfeeding without any difficulties. The baby weighs 10 lb 4 oz and is 23 inches long with a head circumference in the 50th percentile. A 0.5-cm red circular birthmark is noted on the child's left anterior thigh consistent with a port-wine stain. Tiny white facial papules are noted across the nose.

1. Fill in the collected data from this scenario using the documentation tool below.

   Birth History (for the mother of the child)

   Did you receive prenatal care? _____

   How much weight did you gain during pregnancy? _____ lb

   Describe any complications during the pregnancy:

   _____

   Did you use any medications, alcohol, drugs, or herbal/complementary medicines during pregnancy?

   _____ (If yes, list type, amount, and frequency)

   Describe your labor and delivery:

   _____

   How many weeks' gestation was your child born at? _____ weeks

   Describe your child's health immediately after delivery:

   _____

   Is your child breastfed or formula fed?

   _____

2. State the purpose of the birth history from the mother during the well-baby visit:

   _____

   _____

3. List four pieces of objective data that have been collected in this scenario:

   1. _____
   2. _____
   3. _____
   4. _____

4. In the space provided, use a narrative format to document the assessment findings of the skin lesions noted.

   _____

   _____

   _____

OBTAINING DATA

Read the dialogue below and then answer the questions that follow in the space provided.

The following dialogue is between a nurse and a client being admitted to a medical-surgical floor for cellulitis of the left leg.

Nurse: "Mr. Johnson, do you take any medications on a regular basis?"

Client: "I do take a blood pressure pill when I need it."

Nurse: "How do you know when you need your blood pressure pill?"

Client: "I can tell I need it when I start to get a headache and feel very stressed."

Nurse: "How many times per week do you take the pill?"

Client: "Maybe two or three times per week."

Nurse: "What are the instructions on the medication bottle?"

Client: "My doctor thinks I should take it every single day, but I don't think that is necessary."

Nurse: "How often do you have your blood pressure checked?"

Client: "About once per month and it's about 150 over 80."

Nurse: "Can you tell me the name and dosage of the medication you take?"

Client: "It's a little green pill. I don't remember the name, but my doctor said it is a low dose."

1. The above information falls under which category of health history data?

2. Explain why it was necessary for the nurse to ask so many questions in this scenario.

3. Complete the following grid using the data collected from the dialogue:

Medication	Dose	Frequency	Duration	Purpose	Effect

4. List any questions the nurse should ask to complete the data collection.

DOCUMENTATION

Collect a health history on your lab partner and document your findings on the following documentation form. (See Box 8.3 in the text for examples of documented data.)

HEALTH HISTORY

Date: _____

Name: _____

Address: _____

_____

Telephone: _____

Age: _____

Date of Birth: _____

Birthplace: _____

Gender: _____

Marital Status: _____

Race: _____

Religion: _____

Occupation: _____

Health Insurance: _____

_____

Source: _____

Reliability: _____

PRESENT HEALTH/ILLNESS

Reason for seeking care: _____

_____

Height/Weight: _____

Vital Signs:

B/P- _____

HR- _____

RR- _____

T- _____

Allergies: _____

_____

Health Beliefs and Practices: _____

_____

Health Patterns: _____

_____

Medications: _____

_____

Health Goals: _____

PAST HISTORY

Childhood Illnesses: _____

_____

Immunizations: _____

_____

Medical Illnesses: _____

_____

Hospitalizations: _____

_____

Surgery: _____

_____

Injury: _____

Blood Transfusion: _____

Emotional/Psychiatric Problems: _____

_____

Use of Tobacco? _____

Type? Amount? _____

Use of Alcohol? _____

Type? Amount? _____

Use of Illicit Drugs? _____

Type? Amount? _____

FAMILY HISTORY

Father: _____

Mother: _____

Siblings: _____

Grandparents: _____

PSYCHOSOCIAL HISTORY

Occupational History: _____

Educational Level: _____

Financial Background: _____

Roles and Relationships: _____

Ethnicity and Culture: _____

Family: _____

Spirituality: _____

Self-Concept: _____

REVIEW OF SYSTEMS

Skin, Hair, Nails: _____

Head, Neck, Related Lymphatics: _____

Eyes: _____

Ears, Nose, Mouth, and Throat: _____

Respiratory:

_____

Breasts and Axillae: _____

Cardiovascular: _____

Peripheral Vascular: _____

Abdomen: _____

Urinary: _____

Reproductive: _____

Sexual: _____

Musculoskeletal: _____

Neurologic: _____

NCLEX®-STYLE REVIEW QUESTIONS

Read each question carefully. Choose the best answer for each question.

1. A client is injured after falling from a ladder. The best question for the nurse to include when attempting to gather more details about a client's injuries would be:
   1. "Did you fall on concrete?"
   2. "Do you think you broke any bones?"
   3. "Can you describe how you landed when you fell off the ladder?"
   4. "Are you having any pain now?"

2. When obtaining a nutritional history from a 10-year-old, it is best to:
   1. direct the questions to the parents or caregiver
   2. direct the questions to the child
   3. separate the parents or caregiver and the child to question individually and then compare answers for consistency
   4. direct the questions to the child and defer to the parents only when the answer is not known

3. A 16-year-old female is having her annual physical today. What is the best way for the nurse to obtain reliable information regarding sexual history?
   1. Question the girl with her mother present
   2. Ask her to fill out a questionnaire
   3. Question the girl in a private exam room
   4. Omit the sexual history because since she is underage

4. What is the nurse's best action when assessing a young child?
   1. Begin with more invasive or uncomfortable procedures first
   2. Save more invasive or more uncomfortable procedures until last
   3. Avoid using toys, puppets, or other childlike distractors
   4. Avoid letting the child sit on the lap of a parent or caregiver

5. Which client is most likely able to provide the nurse with accurate health history data?
    1. A confused 90-year-old male admitted through the emergency department from a nursing home
    2. A 6-month-old infant who was left in a safe haven crib at a church
    3. A 36-year-old female who arrives at the hospital in active labor
    4. A 76-year-old female who is in a rehabilitation facility for a stroke she had 3 months ago that has left her with expressive aphasia

6. The nurse uses a pictorial display of a client's family relationships and health issues. This is called a:
    1. family tree
    2. pictogram
    3. genealogy
    4. pedigree

7. When obtaining information about a client's medication history, it is important for the nurse to ask the client:
    1. name, purpose, dosage, and the client's understanding of the medication
    2. name, dosage, frequency, and manufacturer of the medication
    3. name, dosage, frequency, and expiration date of the medication
    4. name, purpose, dosage, frequency, duration, and client's understanding of the medication

8. During an interview, a client denies having any medical history. Later, the client states, "I've been taking medication for headaches for 5 years that my doctor gave me." The nurse's response should be:
    1. "Tell me the reason your healthcare provider has prescribed headache medication for you."
    2. "What you are saying to me does not make any sense."
    3. "Why are you taking headache medication?"
    4. "You realize that if you are taking headache medication you have a history of migraines, right?"

9. The nurse questions a client about her sexual orientation. The client states she is attracted to both men and women. What is the most appropriate sexual orientation label the nurse should document?
    1. Gay
    2. Heterosexual
    3. Lesbian
    4. Bisexual

10. The nurse includes which of the following in the review of systems? (Select all that apply.)
    1. Breast and axillae
    2. Emotional history
    3. Reproductive history
    4. Eye history
    5. Smoking history

9 Techniques and Equipment

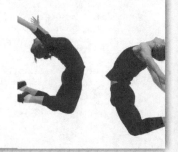

Some men succeed because they are destined to, but most men succeed because they are determined to.

—Greame Clegg

Physical assessment is a process in which the nurse gathers objective and measurable data in order to evaluate a client's overall health status. A systematic approach will assist the nurse in performing an organized assessment. This approach includes four basic techniques: inspection, palpation, percussion, and auscultation. These techniques are used in a repetitive sequence throughout assessment except during abdominal assessment, where the sequence is altered. To enhance the nurse's ability to perform these techniques, various types of equipment may be used. This chapter will review the physical assessment and also safety and comfort measures that should be considered when performing the physical assessment.

OBJECTIVES

At the completion of these exercises, you will be able to:

1. Differentiate between and among the various assessment techniques.
2. Review the purpose of equipment used in the physical assessment.
3. Apply critical thinking in analysis of a case study related to physical assessment.
4. Complete NCLEX®-style review questions related to assessment techniques and equipment.

ASSESSMENT TECHNIQUES

Inspection

Read the following statements regarding the physical assessment technique of inspection. Place a check mark next to each **true** statement. If the statement is not true, rewrite the statement in the space provided so that it accurately reflects the assessment technique of inspection.

_____ 1. Inspection is the first and last technique used in physical assessment.

_____ 2. Inspection begins the moment the nurse meets the client.

_____ 3. Inspection moves from specific details to the general.

_____ 4. Inspection requires bright lighting.

_____ 5. Inspection includes the sense of smell.

_____ 6. Inspection does not require critical thinking skills.

_____ 7. Inspection may determine symmetry.

_____ 8. Inspection should be combined with palpation.

_____ 9. Novice nurses usually feel very comfortable with inspection.

_____ 10. Inspection may require specialty equipment.

Palpation

The following exercise pertains to the assessment technique of palpation. Circle the type of palpation the nurse should use in the assessments identified, then identify which part of the hand the nurse should use to perform the assessment.

1. Lymph nodes

   Light   Moderate   Deep

   Hand surface _____

2. Liver

   Light   Moderate   Deep

   Hand surface _____

3. Skin texture

   Light   Moderate   Deep

   Hand surface _____

4. Skin temperature

   Light   Moderate   Deep

   Hand surface _____

5. Pulses

   Light   Moderate   Deep

   Hand surface _____

6. Fremitus

   Light   Moderate   Deep

   Hand surface _____

Percussion

Part I

The following statements refer to the physical assessment technique of percussion. Using the percussion sounds below, match the appropriate sound to the following statements. Place the letter on the line provided.

T = Tympany   H = Hyperresonance   F = Flatness

R = Resonance   D = Dullness

_____ 1. High-pitched, soft tone of short duration

_____ 2. Low-pitched, loud, hollow tone of long duration

_____ 3. Sound heard when percussing over solid body organs

_____ 4. Sound heard when percussing over air-filled intestines

_____ 5. Sound heard when percussing hyperinflated lungs

_____ 6. High-pitched, loud, drumlike tone of medium duration

_____ 7. Abnormally loud tone of long duration

_____ 8. Sound heard when percussing over bone

_____ 9. Sound heard when percussing over air-filled lungs (normal inflation)

_____ 10. High-pitched, soft tone of short duration

Part II

Label each figure with the correct percussion method (direct, indirect, blunt) and describe the technique in the space provided.

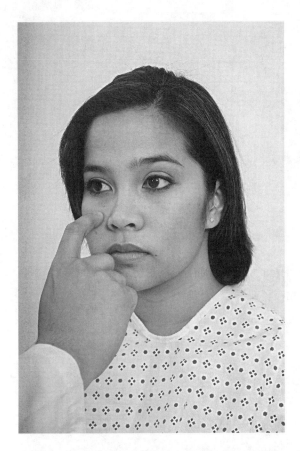

A. _____

_____

_____

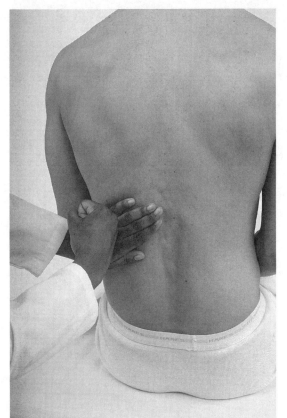

B. _____

_____

_____

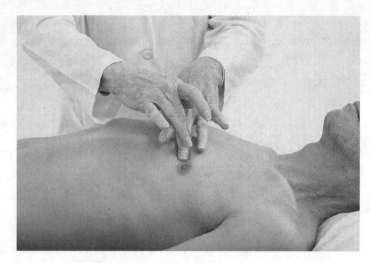

C. _____
   _____
   _____

Part III

Identify the appropriate method of percussion (direct, indirect, blunt) for the following physical assessments.

_____ 1. Maxillary sinuses of a 26-year-old with sinusitis

_____ 2. Posterior thorax to determine diaphragmatic excursion on a 45-year-old

_____ 3. Costovertebral tenderness on a 68-year-old

_____ 4. Borders of the liver on a 19-year-old

_____ 5. Gallbladder tenderness on a 54-year-old

_____ 6. Anterior thorax on a 6-month-old

_____ 7. Frontal sinuses of a 9-year-old

_____ 8. Bladder of a 34-year-old

Auscultation

Part I

The following statements pertain to auscultation. Read each statement, determine if the statement is correct or incorrect, then circle your response. If the statement is incorrect, rewrite the statement correctly.

1. The binaurals of the stethoscope should fit snugly but comfortably.

   Correct   **Incorrect**

   Correction: _____

2. Long stethoscope tubing produces a clearer sound than short tubing.

   Correct   **Incorrect**

   Correction: _____

3. The diaphragm or bell of the stethoscope should be held between the fourth and fifth fingers and placed on the client's chest.

   Correct   **Incorrect**

   Correction: _____

4. The diaphragm should be used to auscultate low-pitched sounds.

   Correct   **Incorrect**

   Correction: _____

5. When auscultating body sounds it is acceptable to place the stethoscope over a client's gown or clothing as long as it is a thin, flat material.

   Correct   **Incorrect**

   Correction:_____

6. The bell should be used to auscultate heart sounds only.

   Correct   **Incorrect**

   Correction: _____

7. Lung sounds obtained by placing the stethoscope on a hair-covered chest require no further assessment.

   Correct   **Incorrect**

   Correction: _____

8. It is best to use a smaller diaphragm and bell when auscultating the body sounds of a child.

   Correct   **Incorrect**

   Correction: _____

9. Heavy pressure should be applied to the skin when using a Doppler ultrasonic stethoscope to obtain pulses.

   Correct   **Incorrect**

   Correction: _____

10. A water-soluble transmission gel should be used with the Doppler ultrasonic stethoscope.

    Correct   **Incorrect**

    Correction: _____

Part II

Identify the sounds below that are detected with a stethoscope. Place a "D" for diaphragm or a "B" for bell on the line provided to indicate which part of the stethoscope the nurse would use in order to best assess the sound. If the sound does not require the use of a stethoscope to be detected, leave the blank empty.

_____   1. Dry, hacking cough

_____   2. Faint expiratory wheeze

_____   3. Dorsalis pedis pulse

_____   4. Bowel sounds

_____   5. Tympany of the abdomen

_____   6. Hoarseness of the voice

_____   7. Heart murmur

_____   8. Carotid bruit

_____   9. Clicking of the temporomandibular joint

_____   10. Apical pulse

_____   11. Pleural friction rub

_____   12. Resonance

EQUIPMENT

Match each piece of equipment in Column A with its appropriate use from Column B. Items in column B are to be used only once.

Column A

_____ 1. Cotton-tipped swab

_____ 2. Gloves

_____ 3. Goggles

_____ 4. Goniometer

_____ 5. Nasal speculum

_____ 6. Ophthalmoscope

_____ 7. Otoscope

_____ 8. Penlight

_____ 9. Reflex hammer

_____ 10. Bell of the stethoscope

_____ 11. Sphygmomanometer

_____ 12. Diaphragm of the stethoscope

_____ 13. Thermometer

_____ 14. Tongue blade

_____ 15. Tuning fork

_____ 16. Vision chart

Column B

A. provides a direct light source and tests pupillary reaction

B. may be used to obtain specimens

C. tests deep tendon reflexes

D. measures body temperature

E. inspection of the external ear and tympanic membrane

F. facilitates examination of the oropharyngeal cavity

G. measures the degree of joint flexion and extension

H. offers eye protection from splashing of body fluids

I. auscultation of heart murmur

J. dilates nares

K. auscultation of lung sounds

L. inspection of the interior structures of the eye

M. assessment of sensation and auditory function

N. protects the client and nurse from contamination

O. screening near and distant vision

P. measures systolic and diastolic blood pressure

APPLICATION OF THE CRITICAL THINKING PROCESS

Read the following scenario and answer the questions as you go along.

Sarah is a registered nurse who works in a women's health clinic. This morning, Gloria, a 26-year-old female, is scheduled for a physical assessment.

1. Name three ways Sarah can prepare a safe and comfortable environment for the client during the physical assessment.

   a.

   b.

   c.

When Sarah first walks into the examination room, she notices that Gloria does not make eye contact with her. Gloria is wearing the examination gown and a pair of dirty, mismatched socks. As Sarah begins to interview the client, she notes that Gloria only provides one- to two-word responses.

2. Identify three observations in this scenario that the nurse should investigate further.

   a.

   b.

   c.

The first thing that Sarah does when she begins the physical assessment is place her stethoscope on Gloria's posterior thorax in order to auscultate her lung sounds. She then has Gloria lay flat in order to palpate and percuss her abdomen. When percussing the abdomen she pays close attention to ensure her motion is coming from the forearm and not the wrist. Sarah uses two strikes before repositioning the pleximeter to avoid muffled sounds. Upon completing the assessment, Sarah washes her hands and informs Gloria that there are some areas in the assessment she feels are abnormal.

   3. Name at least three mistakes that Sarah made during this physical assessment. For each mistake, write how she can improve her technique.

      a. Mistake:

        Correction:

      b. Mistake:

        Correction:

      c. Mistake:

        Correction:

DOCUMENTATION

Complete the following documentation form with your lab partner.

TECHNIQUES AND EQUIPMENT

Name: _____ Date: _____

Age: _____ Gender: _____ Height: _____ Weight: _____

Allergies (medications/food/latex/other): _____

Growth and developmental considerations: _____

FOCUSED INTERVIEW (SUBJECTIVE DATA)

Reason for today's visit: _____

_____

Past medical history: _____ Surgeries: _____

General health: _____

Cultural/religious/psychosocial considerations: _____

PHYSICAL ASSESSMENT (OBJECTIVE DATA)

Inspection

General survey of patient's appearance (survey general overview, then specific detail):

_____

Body parts symmetrical?

_____

For each body system, note color, size, shape, contour, symmetry, movement, drainage, odor:

_____

Any abnormal findings noted? Yes/No. If yes, describe:

_____

Palpation

For each body system, which technique used? Light/Moderate/Deep palpation
Note size, shape, location, mobility of a part, position, vibrations, temperature, texture, moisture, tenderness, or edema:

_____

_____

Note which part of hand used (finger pads, fingertips, palmar surface of fingers or hands, ulnar surface, or dorsal surface):

_____

Any abnormal findings noted? Yes/No. If yes, describe:

_____

Any pain or discomfort reported?

_____

Percussion

For each body system, which technique used? Direct/Blunt/Indirect
Type of sound:

     Tympany? _____

     Resonance? _____

     Hyperresonance? _____

     Dullness? _____

     Flatness? _____

       *Note location, intensity, pitch, duration, and quality of each sound.

Any abnormal findings noted? Yes/No. If yes, describe:

_____

Any pain or discomfort reported?

_____

Auscultation

For appropriate body system, note if the bell or diaphragm used: _____

Description of sound

     Intensity: _____

     Pitch: _____

     Duration: _____

     Quality: _____

Absence of expected sound? Yes/No. If yes, describe:

_____

Any pain or discomfort reported?

_____

Equipment

Note any equipment used during the physical assessment, including, but not limited to: computer, cotton balls, cotton-tipped applicators, culture media, dental mirror, flashlight, gauze, gloves, goggles, lubricant, speculums, reflex hammer, ruler, scale, marking pen, slides, specimen containers, sphygmomanometer, stadiometer, tape measure, test tubes, thermometer, tongue blade, tuning fork, vision chart, watch with second hand.

Stethoscope

Diaphragm or bell used?

Blood pressure:

Heart sounds:

Respirations:

Bowel sounds:

Doppler ultrasonic stethoscope

Fetal heart rate:

Peripheral pulses:

Ophthalmoscope

Any abnormal findings? Pallor or hemorrhaging?

Lesions? Describe:

Otoscope

Describe any abnormal external or internal ear structures:

Special equipment
Goniometer

Degree of flexion or extension:

Skinfold calipers

Subcutaneous tissue thickness:

Transilluminator

Blood, fluid, or masses detected?

Wood's lamp

Presence of fungal infection?

Special Considerations
Patients with obesity:

Adequate sized chairs/beds?

Secured examination table or locked hospital bed?

Appropriate scale?

Large blood pressure cuff available?

Standard precautions:

Frequent hand washing?

Gloves worn?

Sharps container available?

Appropriate cleaning or disposal of equipment?

Patient safety ensured at all times?

NCLEX®-STYLE REVIEW QUESTIONS

Read each question carefully. Choose the best answer for each question.

1. Which of the following sequences used during physical assessment reflects the proper order for the nurse to assess a client?
   1. Auscultation, percussion, palpation, inspection
   2. Inspection, percussion, palpation, auscultation
   3. Inspection, palpation, percussion, auscultation
   4. Palpation, inspection, percussion, auscultation

2. A young adult is involved in a motorcycle crash and sustains injuries to the right leg. As the nurse inspects the client's injured leg, it is best to proceed from:
   1. distal to proximal and then to the entire leg
   2. proximal to distal and then to the entire leg
   3. the entire leg and then distal to proximal
   4. the entire leg and then proximal to distal

3. The nurse uses _____ percussion when assessing the thorax of an infant.
   1. indirect
   2. blunt
   3. direct
   4. deep

4. When using the ophthalmoscope to inspect the interior structures of the eye, the nurse identifies an abnormal finding. The best aperture to use to further assess a lesion would be a:
   1. small aperture
   2. slit
   3. grid
   4. red-free filter

5. Two agencies that help to establish protocols to protect both nurses and clients from the spread of disease are:
   1. the Centers for Disease Control and the Occupational Safety and Health Administration
   2. the American Nurses Association and the American Medical Association
   3. the Centers for Disease Control and the American Nurses Association
   4. the American Medical Association and the Occupational Safety and Health Administration

6. A nursing student is performing a physical assessment in the clinical setting. The nursing instructor provides further teaching when the student:
   1. performs hand hygiene only at the beginning of the assessment
   2. cleanses the bell and diaphragm of the stethoscope with disinfectant prior to applying it on a client
   3. carefully inspects a body part before palpating the area
   4. wears gloves if there is any potential for exposure to blood or body fluids

7. The nurse is preparing to assess the fetal heart rate of a client who is 5 months pregnant using a Doppler ultrasonic stethoscope. The nurse understands in order to accurately obtain the fetal heart rate, it is important to:
   1. use a transducer gel
   2. use heavy pressure
   3. cool the transducer before touching the client's skin
   4. have the client exhale and then hold her breath

8. The nurse is palpating the peripheral pulses of an older adult client. Important factors for the nurse to consider when performing this type of assessment are: (Select all that apply.)
   1. making certain fingernails are short and smooth
   2. not wearing jewelry
   3. assessing the client for a latex allergy
   4. performing hand hygiene before and after assessment
   5. putting on sterile gloves for the assessment

9. The nurse is assessing the abdomen of a client who may be infected with hepatitis B. In order to assess for hepatomegaly, the nurse will palpate:
    1. less than 1 cm deep over the left upper quadrant
    2. 2–4 cm deep over the left upper quadrant
    3. less than 1 cm deep over the right upper quadrant
    4. 2–4 cm deep over the right upper quadrant

10. The nurse is caring for an adult client weighing >400 lb. Which blood pressure cuff is most appropriate to measure the blood pressure on this client's arm?
    1. An extra-large adult-sized cuff
    2. A thigh cuff
    3. Cuff with bladder width of 40% to 50% of arm circumference
    4. A palpated systolic pressure should be measured

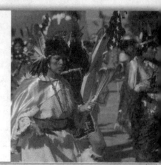

10 › General Survey

The undertaking of a new action brings new strength.
—Richard L. Evans

The general survey begins when the nurse first sees the client. This "first impression" requires education, skillful use of the senses to recognize clues and gather information, and knowledge to quickly analyze the data to determine the appropriate approach for the physical assessment. Some may call the ability to create a first impression a sixth sense; however, with education and practice you will learn how to focus on important observations during the first few minutes spent with the client. This chapter will review and apply the knowledge learned about the general survey and the measurement of vital signs.

OBJECTIVES

At the completion of these exercises, you will be able to:

1. Categorize observations as part of the general survey.
2. Identify appropriate routes for measuring body temperatures.
3. Identify the location of peripheral pulses.
4. Review the proper sequence for obtaining a blood pressure.
5. Recognize factors that influence vital signs.
6. Perform a general survey.
7. Obtain a full set of vital signs.
8. Prioritize scenarios based on general survey observations.
9. Document data collected during a general survey.
10. Apply the critical thinking process to case studies related to the general survey.
11. Complete NCLEX®-style review questions related to the general survey.

ROUTES FOR MEASURING TEMPERATURE

List the five routes for measuring core body temperature. Then identify a situation in which this route would be contraindicated.

1. _____

   Contraindication: _____

2. _____

   Contraindication: _____

3. _____

   Contraindication: _____

4. _____

   Contraindication: _____

5. _____

   Contraindication: _____

PULSE LOCATIONS

On the line provided write the name of the pulse described in each of the statements. Locate the pulse on the diagram by placing the number on the line matching the anatomic position of the pulse.

1. Pulse locations

    1. Located between the eye and the top of the ear _____

    2. Located halfway between the anterior superior iliac spine and the symphysis pubis _____

    3. Located behind and slightly inferior to the medial malleolus

       _____

    4. Located in the popliteal fossa lateral to the midline _____

    5. Located on the thumb side of the anterior wrist _____

    6. Located in the medial aspect of the antecubital fossa _____

    7. Located in the groove between the trachea and the sternocleidomastoid

       _____

    8. Located on the medial side of the dorsum of the foot _____

2. Explain the steps the nurse may take if she is unable to palpate a pedal pulse.

    _____

    _____

    _____

RESPIRATIONS

Read each statement and decide whether it is true or false. Circle your answer. If the answer is false, rewrite the statement to make it true.

1. Each inspiration should be counted independently of each expiration.

    True   **False**

    _____

2. A respiratory rate of 52 respirations per minute for a newborn is a normal finding.

    True   **False**

    _____

3. The nurse should count a respiratory rate for one full minute at all times.

    True   **False**

    _____

4. To obtain accurate data, the nurse should not inform the client that he is counting respirations.

    True   **False**

    _____

5. A respiratory rate of 30 (26 is a trivial value) respirations per minute for a 6-year-old is an abnormal finding.

   True   **False**

   _____

6. Medications may alter a client's respiratory rate.

   True   **False**

   _____

7. A full respiratory cycle contains one inspiration and one expiration.

   True   **False**

   _____

8. A respiratory rate of 8 is considered a normal finding in the older adult.

   True   **False**

   _____

BLOOD PRESSURE

Place the following steps for measuring a client's blood pressure in the correct order from 1 (the first step) through 15 (the last step).

_____   Palpate the brachial pulse.

_____   Place the client in a comfortable position.

_____   Deflate the cuff rapidly and completely.

_____   Place the diaphragm of the stethoscope over the brachial pulse.

_____   Palpate the radial pulse.

_____   Remove any clothing from the client's arm.

_____   Confirm that the blood pressure cuff is the appropriate size for the client's arm.

_____   Note the manometer reading at each of the five Korotkoff phases.

_____   Close the release valve on the pump.

_____   Remove the cuff from the client's arm.

_____   Slightly flex the arm and hold it at the level of the heart with the palm upward.

_____   Pump up the cuff until the sphygmomanometer registers 30 mmHg above the palpatory systolic blood pressure.

_____   Place the cuff on the arm with the lower border 1 inch above the antecubital area, making sure that the cuff is smooth and snug.

_____   Inflate the cuff until the radial pulse is no longer palpable and note the reading on the sphygmomanometer.

_____   Release the valve on the cuff carefully so that the pressure decreases at the rate of 2 to 3 mmHg per second.

FACTORS THAT INFLUENCE VITAL SIGNS

Read each statement. Circle the anticipated change for the stated vital sign discussed in the statement.

1. A male who has stepped off the treadmill after running 7 miles

   Temperature   Lower   No Change   Higher

2. A preschool child who has a fever of 103.6°F

   Respirations   Lower   No Change   Higher

3. An adolescent 14 days into her 28-day menstrual cycle

   Temperature   Lower   No Change   Higher

4. A middle-aged adult who is nervous about scheduled surgery

   Blood Pressure   Lower   No Change   Higher

5. A school-age child who has a fever of 104.2°F

   Pulse   Lower   No Change   Higher

6. A young adult who has climbed to the top of Mount Everest

   Respirations   Lower   No Change   Higher

7. An older adult who has just returned to his hospital room after a physical therapy session

   Pulse   Lower   No Change   Higher

8. A client who has just received an injection of morphine to relieve her postoperative pain

   Blood Pressure   Lower   No Change   Higher

9. A young adult who is giving a presentation to 1000 people at work that he just finished preparing 1 hour ago

   Temperature   Lower   No Change   Higher

10. An adolescent client who has lost 400 ml of blood from her abdominal incision reopening

    Pulse   Lower   No Change   Higher

11. A middle-age adult who is anxious about his upcoming colonoscopy

    Respirations   Lower   No Change   Higher

12. An older adult who is meditating

    Blood Pressure   Lower   No Change   Higher

13. A middle-age adult who has gained 100 lb in the past 10 years

    Blood Pressure   Lower   No Change   Higher

14. An adolescent who is shoveling snow

    Respirations   Lower   No Change   Higher

15. A 3-year-old child hospitalized for hypothermia

    Oxygen Saturation   Lower   No Change   Higher

APPLICATION OF THE CRITICAL THINKING PROCESS

Read each general survey scenario. Identify which client is the first priority to be evaluated based on your observations. Provide a rationale for your answer.

_____ A 75-year-old male who is sitting in a wheelchair, skin color pale. Client is in no apparent distress. Client is wearing clean, warm clothing.

Vital signs: BP 168/102 – HR 112 – RR 16 – Temp 98.2

_____ A 26-year-old female who is sitting with her head leaning over into her lap, skin color is pink. She is dressed appropriately for the weather. Her body frame is large and she appears overweight.

Vital Signs: BP 122/84 – HR 110 – RR 18 – Temp 102.4

_____ A 56-year-old male who is unresponsive with agonal breathing, skin color pallor with bluish undertones.

Vital Signs: BP 68/42 – HR 42 – RR 4 – Temp 96.2

_____ A 15-year-old female who limps in the doorway wearing a cheerleading uniform, skin color pink. She sits down slowly and moves a chair to raise her left leg and places an ice pack to her ankle. She is laughing with the people who accompanied her in and is eating a bag of chips.

Vital Signs: BP 110/62 – HR 76 – RR 16 – Temp 98.1

_____ A 66-year-old male grabbing at his chest and moaning in pain. His skin color is pink. He is morbidly obese and wearing pajama pants and a T-shirt that appears to have vomit on it.

Vital Signs: BP 168/92 – HR 86 – RR 24 – Temp 99.7

First Priority

Rationale: _____

_____

_____

Read the scenario below and then answer the questions that follow in the space provided.

Allison is a 32-year-old female who arrives at an urgent care center stating "my stomach has been killing me since last night." She is sitting in a chair using her arms to hold her abdomen as she rocks back and forth. She is dressed in a long, blue velvet gown with a tiara on her head. As you move closer to her, you note the smell of cigarette smoke. She is about 5′2″ and 120 lbs. When you speak to her, she replies with short answers and makes facial grimaces.

1. Identify at least four observations made regarding the general survey.

    1.

    2.

    3.

    4.

You begin to gather more data and decide to continue by measuring her vital signs. You decide to measure an oral temperature. The temperature reading is 101.2°F. Her blood pressure reading is 116/72. Her right radial pulse is 122 bpm and feels weak. Next you obtain the respiratory rate, which is 18 respirations per minute. The oxygen saturation is 99% on room air.

2. Sort the data identified as a normal or abnormal finding.

    Normal   **Abnormal**

DOCUMENTATION

Perform a general survey and obtain a complete set of vital signs on your lab partner and document your findings on the following documentation form.

Today's Date: _____

GENERAL SURVEY
Client Name: _____
Date of Birth: _____
Gender: _____

Physical Appearance:
    Facial symmetry: _____
    Skin color: _____
    Hair: _____
    Height: _____ Weight: _____

Mental Status:
    Oriented to person/place/date/purpose? _____
    Affect and generalized mood: _____
    Level of anxiety: _____
    Speech (clear, slurred, coherent…?): _____

Mobility:
    Gait: _____
    Posture: _____
    Range of motion: _____

Behavior:
    Dress and grooming: _____
    Body odors: _____
    Facial expression: _____
    Ability to make eye contact: _____

VITAL SIGNS
BP: _____ Site: _____
HR: _____
RR: _____
Temp: _____ Route: _____
O_2 saturation: _____ Oxygen/room air: _____

NCLEX®-STYLE REVIEW QUESTIONS

Read each question carefully. Choose the best answer for each question.

1. The nurse is aware that the four major categories of the general survey are:
    1. physical appearance, mental status, mobility, and behavior
    2. physical appearance, mental status, cognitive function, and vital signs
    3. physical appearance, cognitive function, height-versus-weight ratio, and vital signs
    4. mental status, cognitive function, mobility, and behavior

2. The nurse assessing the heart rate of a 5-month-old baby knows the most appropriate place to assess is the:
    1. radial pulse
    2. carotid pulse
    3. apical pulse
    4. brachial pulse

3. The nurse is counting the respiratory rate of a client experiencing an acute asthma attack. The nurse knows that in order to obtain an accurate count he should:
    1. count each inspiration and expiration separately
    2. count the number of breaths for 30 seconds and then multiply by 2
    3. not inform the client that he is counting a respiratory rate
    4. estimate the rate and document tachypnea in the client record

4. A 32-year-old female, with a large frame, has a height of 5′8″ and a weight of 175 lb. The nurse concludes that:
    1. this is an appropriate weight for her height and large frame
    2. this is underweight for her height and large frame
    3. this is overweight for her height and large frame
    4. the client is morbidly obese

5. The nurse obtains an oxygen saturation level on an adult client as 97%. The nurse concludes that this reading is:
    1. within a normal range
    2. less than expected
    3. life threatening
    4. The oxygen saturation level is not measured in percentages

6. A young adult client has been monitoring her body temperature to determine when she is ovulating. She measures her oral temperature every morning when she awakens at 6:30 a.m. Each day the thermometer reads 98.2°F. What reading would indicate ovulation?
    1. 97.2°F
    2. 96°F
    3. 98.7°F
    4. 101°F

7. The nurse is aware that the following factors can affect a client's blood pressure. (Select all that apply.)
    1. Obesity
    2. Gender
    3. Diurnal variations
    4. Medications
    5. Physical activity

8. When auscultating a blood pressure, the nurse identifies the Korotkoff sounds. When listening for these sounds, the nurse is able to determine the blood pressure by documenting:
    1. phase 1 as the systolic pressure and phase 5 as the diastolic pressure
    2. phase 1 as the systolic pressure and the number just before phase 4 begins as the diastolic pressure
    3. the number at the beginning of phase 2 as the systolic pressure and the end of phase 4 as the diastolic pressure
    4. the number at the beginning of phase 2 as the systolic pressure and the end of phase 5 as the diastolic pressure

9. A 19-year-old female presents to the clinic on a hot summer day for her annual exam. While she sits in the waiting area she is wearing dark sunglasses and a long-sleeve shirt. As her name is called she walks slowly into the examination room with her head down. When she sits down on the table you obtain a full set of vital signs and begin to ask her health history questions. The first piece of assessment data collected in this scenario would be:
   1. the vital signs
   2. the health history
   3. her physical appearance
   4. The assessment has not begun yet

10. The nurse is unable to obtain a pulse oximetry reading on the finger probe of a client who suffered major blood loss. What is the nurse's best action?
    1. Place probe on the great toe
    2. Notify the healthcare provider
    3. Document pulse oximetry was not obtained
    4. Place the probe on the client's earlobe

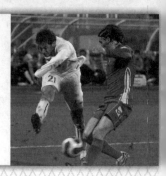

11 Pain Assessment

We cannot learn without pain.
—Aristotle

Pain is unique and has a different meaning to each individual. Each painful experience, combined with one's psychosocial background, brings a different response. The nurse must be able to perform an accurate pain assessment in order to develop an individualized plan of care for the client. This chapter will provide you with an understanding of various types of pain and assist in developing the skill of performing a pain assessment utilizing various tools.

OBJECTIVES

At the completion of these exercises, you will be able to:

1. Differentiate between acute and chronic pain.
2. Categorize various types of pain.
3. Explore pain assessment tools.
4. Identify factors that may influence a person's pain perception.
5. Perform and document a pain assessment.
6. Complete NCLEX®-style review questions related to the pain assessment.

PAIN ASSESSMENT ACRONYMS

Pain is the fifth vital sign. List the components of the pain assessment using the following acronyms.

O: _____

L: _____

D: _____

C: _____

A: _____

R: _____

T: _____

I: _____

C: _____

E: _____

ACUTE VERSUS CHRONIC PAIN

1. Review the characteristics of pain listed below. Place the letter that corresponds with each characteristic in the appropriate circle. Use each letter only once.

Characteristics

A. Prolonged over 6 months
B. Lasts only through recovery period
C. Client reports pain
D. Client often doesn't mention pain
E. Sympathetic nervous system response

F. Parasympathetic nervous system response
G. Restless and anxious client
H. Depressed and withdrawn client

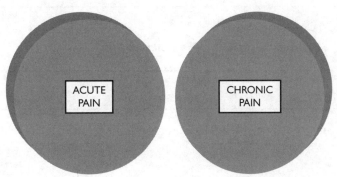

2. Identify the pain associated with each of the problems below as acute or chronic by writing an **"A"** for acute or a **"C"** for chronic on the line provided.

_____ 1. Ruptured appendix

_____ 2. Pancreatic cancer

_____ 3. Fibromyalgia

_____ 4. Laceration to left third digit

_____ 5. Childbirth

_____ 6. Fractured hip

_____ 7. Rheumatoid arthritis

_____ 8. Myocardial infarction

_____ 9. Inguinal hernia

_____ 10. Degenerative disc disease

_____ 11. Ischemic colon

_____ 12. Renal calculi

From above, select one acute pain problem and one chronic pain problem and provide a rationale for your classification.

Acute pain:

_____

_____

Chronic pain:

_____

_____

CATEGORIES OF PAIN

Circle the most appropriate descriptor for each type of pain. Write the rationale for your answer on the line provided.

1. Torn anterior cruciate ligament

   Cutaneous pain   **Deep somatic pain**   **Visceral pain**

   Rationale: _____

2. Abrasions to the right arm

   Intractable pain   **Neuropathic pain**   **Cutaneous pain**

   Rationale: _____

3. Osteosarcoma

   Radiating pain   **Visceral pain**   **Cutaneous pain**

   Rationale: _____

4. Herpes zoster

   Neuropathic pain   **Intractable pain**   **Referred pain**

   Rationale: _____

5. Client report of pain in a leg that has been surgically amputated

   Intractable pain   **Radiating pain**   **Phantom pain**

   Rationale: _____

6. Right shoulder pain from cholecystitis

   Intractable pain   **Neuropathic pain**   **Referred pain**

   Rationale: _____

PAIN ASSESSMENT TOOLS

1. Draw an example of the Numeric Rating Scale in the space provided.

2. Answer the following questions referring to various pain scales.

   1. Which pain scale would be the most appropriate to use with a 5-year-old? Explain your answer.

   2. You are about to use the Simple Verbal Descriptive Scale to assess the pain intensity of your client. In the space provided below, describe how you would introduce this scale to your client in order to obtain accurate data.

3. Use a nursing database to research the FLACC scale.

   a. What database did you use?

   b. In the space below, write what each letter stands for.

      F—

      L—

      A—

      C—

      C—

   c. Explain how this scale is scored.

APPLICATION OF THE CRITICAL THINKING PROCESS

Read the scenario below and then answer the questions that follow in the space provided.

Mr. Pineapple (white Anglo-Saxon) and Mrs. Wong (Chinese) have each had a total hip replacement. Mr. Pineapple has a client-controlled analgesic pump (PCA) and is receiving a small dose of morphine every 10 minutes. He rates his pain as an 8 on a numerical scale of 0 to 10. Mrs. Wong refused the morphine pump and prefers to use over-the-counter Motrin for the pain. She rates her pain as a 3 on a numerical scale of 0 to 10.

1. Which client is experiencing the greater amount of pain? Explain your answer.

2. Explain how two people who have had the same surgery can experience different levels of pain.

FACTORS INFLUENCING PAIN ASSESSMENT

Read the following scenario and answer the questions as you go along.

Ms. Lemon is a 56-year-old female who was diagnosed with stomach cancer 18 months ago. She has undergone a partial gastrectomy (removal of the stomach) accompanied by radiation and chemotherapy for 6 months. She has recently been informed her cancer has metastasized to her liver. She has been experiencing pain for months. Her past history includes herniated discs from L4–S1, cholecystectomy, appendectomy, total knee replacement, and three caesarean sections.

1. Is Ms. Lemon experiencing acute pain or chronic pain? Provide a rationale for your decision.

Ms. Lemon comes to the outpatient infusion center for her chemotherapy. Prior to connecting Ms. Lemon to her chemotherapy infusion, you must complete a pain assessment. You ask her the following questions:

Where is your pain located?

Can you rate your pain on a scale of 0–10, with 0 being no pain and 10 being the worst pain imaginable?

Is the pain constant or intermittent?

2. List four additional questions that should be asked during this assessment.

   1.

   2.

   3.

   4.

Ms. Lemon states that her body constantly aches all over. A few times per day she gets a sharp pressure pain in her upper abdomen. She states her pain fluctuates from a 3 to an 8 on a scale of 0–10. She is using an opioid skin patch for pain that she changes every 3 days and is also taking OxyContin twice per day. She seems confused about the medications she is taking and fears that she will die from the medication and not the cancer.

3. You decide to develop a teaching plan for Ms. Lemon. In the space below, write one goal that would be important to achieve.

4. Write two objectives that would support your goal.

   1.

   2.

5. Explain how you would evaluate each objective.

   1.

   2.

DOCUMENTATION

Perform a pain assessment on your lab partner and document your findings on the following documentation form.

PAIN HISTORY

Vital Signs: BP _____ HR _____ RR _____ Temp _____ O$_2$ sat _____

*Use quotation marks to record the description of the pain in the exact words of the client for the following questions.

ONSET

1. When did the pain begin?
2. Can you describe any circumstances associated with the onset of pain?

LOCATION

1. Where is your pain?
2. Does the pain move or is it just in one place?
3. Are you able to point to or put your finger on the painful area?

DURATION

1. Do you have pain now?
2. Is the pain constant or intermittent?
3. How long does the pain last?

CHARACTERISTICS of the Pain

1. How bad is the pain now?
2. Using a scale of 0–10, with 0 being no pain and 10 being the worst possible pain, how would you rate your present pain level?
3. An alternative method would be to give the patient a pain intensity scale (refer to Figure 11.7).
4. What does the pain feel like?
5. Describe your pain.
6. An alternative method would be to list the possible descriptive terms and ask the patient to respond "yes" or "no" to each descriptor.

AGGRAVATING Factors

1. What do you think started the pain?
2. What were you doing just before the pain started?
3. Have you been under a great deal of stress lately?
4. An added method to determine aggravating factors is to list common factors and ask the patient to respond "yes" or "no" when the list is read. The factors would include but are not limited to moving, walking, turning, breathing, swallowing, and urinating.

RELIEVING Factors

1. What have you done to relieve the pain?
2. Did it work?
3. Have you used this before? When?
4. Why do you think it worked (or did not work) this time?

TREATMENT

1. Do you take a prescribed pain pill?
2. Do you take an over-the-counter medicine for the pain?
3. Do you change your diet in any way when you have pain?
4. Do you use an ice pack or heating pad on the pain?
5. Do you use prayer?
6. Do you or a family member perform some ritual?
7. Do you rest when you have the pain?
8. Do you do anything that has not been mentioned?

IMPACT on Activities of Daily Living (ADLs)

1. Describe your daily activities.
2. How well are you able to perform these activities?
3. Does the pain in any way hinder your ability to function?
4. An alternative method would be to list possible daily activities and ask the patient to respond with a "yes" or "no" if the pain hinders the ability to perform the actions.

COPING Strategies

1. Describe how you deal or cope with the pain.
2. Are you in a support group for pain?
3. What do you do to decrease the pain so you can function and feel better?

EMOTIONAL Responses

1. Emotionally, how does the pain make you feel?
2. Does your pain make you feel depressed?
3. Does your pain ever make you feel anxious, tired, or exhausted?

Describe any physiologic or nonverbal responses to pain:

1. Facial expression
2. Vocalizations (moaning, crying, etc.)
3. Immobilization of affected body part
4. Purposeless body movements (ex: involuntary jerking, tossing and turning, etc.)
5. Rhythmic body movements
6. Vital sign and nervous system changes (ex: diaphoresis, increased blood pressure, etc.)

NCLEX®-STYLE REVIEW QUESTIONS

Read each question carefully. Choose the best answer for each question.

1. The nurse understands that pain is:
    1. subjective
    2. objective
    3. a similar experience for persons undergoing similar injuries, illnesses, and treatments
    4. dependent on the nurse's perception of the client's experience

2. The nurse understands that the receptors that transmit pain sensation are called:
    1. modulators
    2. gait controllers
    3. nociceptors
    4. impulse regulators

3. When performing a pain assessment, the nurse must consider which of the following factors? (Select all that apply.)
    1. Psychological factors
    2. Sociocultural factors
    3. Behavioral factors
    4. Environmental factors
    5. Developmental factors

4. The nurse identifies an example of a mechanical stimulus that can excite pain receptors as:
    1. frostbite
    2. renal calculi (kidney stones)
    3. second-degree burn
    4. angina

5. A client is experiencing acute pain. The nurse knows that the sympathetic nervous system will initially respond by:
    1. decreasing the heart rate and blood pressure
    2. constricting the pupils
    3. causing diaphoresis
    4. decreasing the respiratory rate

6. An adult male is brought to an emergency department via ambulance because he was an unrestrained passenger in a motor vehicle crash. He states that he has a high tolerance for pain. The nurse interprets this statement as:
    1. the client has a low pain threshold
    2. the client has a high pain threshold
    3. the client has a limited pain reaction
    4. the pain threshold is not the same as pain tolerance

7. A middle-age Chinese American female arrives at a women's health clinic complaining of a burning sensation when she voids bloody urine. After an examination, the nurse practitioner (NP) explains to the client that she has a very bad urinary tract infection. The NP writes her a prescription for an antibiotic, but the client refuses any pain medication. The nurse is aware that this may be due to:
    1. the client's fear of narcotic addiction
    2. the client's Chinese culture may lead her to be stoic
    3. the minimal pain that is typically experienced with a urinary tract infection doesn't really require pain medication
    4. the client's lack of trust in nurse practitioners

8. A young child is seen with a fractured right radius after falling from a trampoline. The nurse caring for this client knows it is best to:
    1. send the parents to the waiting area so they don't have to see their child in pain
    2. encourage the parents to hold the child to provide comfort
    3. avoid using distraction techniques because it is best to have the child aware of what is going on at all times
    4. use the Numeric Rating Scale to assess the child's pain

9. An older adult who lives in a long-term care facility has become increasingly lethargic in the past 24 hours. The client is transferred from the long-term care facility to the emergency department, where it is determined the client has appendicitis. The nurse recognizes which of the following statements as correct when dealing with pain in the older adult? (Select all that apply.)
    1. Lethargy and fatigue may be an indicator of pain
    2. The older adult may misinterpret pain as part of the aging process
    3. The older adult may have decreased sensations of pain
    4. The prevalence of pain is lower in the older adult population
    5. The older adult requires more pain medication due to physiologic changes associated with aging

10. An adult client suffers from migraine headaches and is seen frequently by the healthcare provider (HCP) for pain management. Which question would be **inappropriate** for the nurse to ask the client during a focused interview regarding pain?
    1. "How bad is the pain now?"
    2. "How long does the pain last?"
    3. "Why are you smiling at me if you're having pain?"
    4. "What were you doing just before the pain started?"

Nutritional Assessment

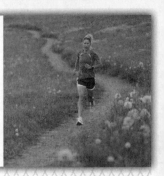

You only get out what you put in.
—Unknown

Nutritional health is a vital component of the overall health status of the individual. Some of the leading causes of death can be caused by poor dietary habits. This includes but is not limited to coronary artery disease and diabetes mellitus. Although nurses work collaboratively with members of other disciplines, such as dietitians and nutritionists, nurses must be capable of performing a nutritional assessment. The data collected will allow the nurse to incorporate dietary changes in the plan of care or make referrals to other disciplines in order to further assess a client's needs.

OBJECTIVES

At the completion of these exercises, you will be able to:

1. Complete a nutritional history.
2. Analyze anthropometric measurements.
3. Identify nutritional deficiencies that may lead to physical findings.
4. Perform and document a nutritional assessment including assessment of cultural diet influences.
5. Evaluate nutritional assessment data.
6. Complete NCLEX®-style review questions related to nutrition.

THE NUTRITIONAL HISTORY

The 24-Hour Diet Recall

Review the following sample 24-hour diet recall. Then, in the space provided on the right, document all the food and beverages you consumed in the past 24 hours.

SAMPLE RECALL		MY PERSONAL RECALL	
TYPE OF FOOD	PORTION	TYPE OF FOOD	PORTION
Cheerios	1 cup		
Skim milk	1 cup		
Banana	1 small		
Orange juice	½ cup		
Almonds, dry roasted, unsalted	¼ cup		
Apple	1 small		
Water	16 oz		
Grilled cheese sandwich			
American cheese	2 slices		
Whole-wheat bread	2 slices		
Tomato	1		
Deli pickle	1 cup		
Herbal tea	8 oz		
Water	16 oz		

SAMPLE RECALL		MY PERSONAL RECALL	
TYPE OF FOOD	PORTION	TYPE OF FOOD	PORTION
Low-fat yogurt	3/4 cup		
Fresh strawberries	1/4 cup		
Water	16 oz		
Grilled chicken	8 oz		
Baked potato	1 small		
Steamed broccoli	1 1/2 cups		
Chocolate pudding	1 cup		
Iced tea	32 oz		

BODY MASS INDEX

Use Table 12.5 in Chapter 12 of the text to determine the body mass index for each client listed. Use the following key to interpret your findings and place the interpretation on the line.

U = Underweight   **H** = Healthy Weight   **OW** = Overweight   **OB** = Obese

_____ _____ 1. 24-year-old female who is 5′ tall and weighs 143 lb

_____ _____ 2. 62-year-old male who is 5′8″ tall and weighs 258 lb

_____ _____ 3. 43-year-old female who is 5′3″ tall and weighs 120 lb

_____ _____ 4. 37-year-old female who is 5′6″ tall and weighs 148 lb

_____ _____ 5. 92-year-old female who is 5′2″ tall and weighs 95 lb

_____ _____ 6. 68-year-old male who is 6′2″ tall and weighs 200 lb

_____ _____ 7. 45-year-old male who is 6′ tall and weighs 175 lb

_____ _____ 8. 55-year-old female who is 5′4″ tall and weighs 220 lb

_____ _____ 9. 18-year-old male who is 5′9″ tall and weighs 175 lb

_____ _____ 10. 57-year-old female who is 4′10″ tall and weighs 85 lb

ASSESSMENT FINDINGS

Identify each piece of data as either "N" for normal or "A" for abnormal by circling the letter below each finding. Write the potential nutritional deficit on the line below each abnormal finding.

1. Bleeding gums

   N   A_____

2. Goiter

   N   A_____

3. Pallor

   N   A_____

4. Tongue midline

   N   A_____

5. Brittle hair

   N   A_____

6. Nail bed curvature of 160°

   N   A_____

7. Pitting edema

N   A _____

8. Bowed legs

N   A _____

9. Freckles

N   A _____

10. Smooth tongue

N   A _____

CHOOSE MY PLATE

Log on to the www.choosemyplate.gov website. (This site has replaced the Food Pyramid by the USDA.) Use the Interactive Tools to develop your own "plate."

1. How many calories are suggested for you per day?

2. List the amount of each food in each group that is suggested.

Grains

Vegetables

Fruits

Dairy

Protein foods

Oils

3. Compare the suggested food selections and portions with your personal 24-hour diet recall from the Nutritional History section at the beginning of this chapter.

1. Which food groups are you meeting appropriately?

2. Which food groups demonstrate a deficiency?

3. Which food groups demonstrate an abundance?

4. Is the 24-hour diet recall the appropriate assessment tool to use for this exercise? If not, which assessment tool would be more appropriate?

5. Develop a 2-day menu that meets the recommended daily amounts of each food group according to MyPlate.gov.

Example	
Breakfast	**Calories** 210
Cheerios 1 cup	
Skim milk 1 cup	**Food Groups**
	Grains
	Milk

DAY 1		DAY 2	
Breakfast	Calories	Breakfast	Calories
	Food Groups		Food Groups
Snack	Calories	Snack	Calories
	Food Groups		Food Groups
Lunch	Calories	Lunch	Calories
	Food Groups		Food Groups
Snack	Calories	Snack	Calories
	Food Groups		Food Groups
Dinner	Calories	Dinner	Calories
	Food Groups		Food Groups

LAB ASSIGNMENT

Complete the Mini Nutritional Assessment (MNA) on another student in your clinical laboratory.

Mini Nutritional Assessment
MNA®

Nestlé Nutrition Institute

Last name:		First name:	
Sex:	Age:	Weight, kg:	Height, cm:	Date:

Complete the screen by filling in the boxes with the appropriate numbers.
Add the numbers for the screen. If score is 11 or less, continue with the assessment to gain a Malnutrition Indicator Score.

Screening

A Has food intake declined over the past 3 months due to loss of appetite, digestive problems, chewing or swallowing difficulties?
0 = severe decrease in food intake
1 = moderate decrease in food intake
2 = no decrease in food intake ☐

B Weight loss during the last 3 months
0 = weight loss greater than 3kg (6.6lbs)
1 = does not know
2 = weight loss between 1 and 3kg (2.2 and 6.6 lbs)
3 = no weight loss ☐

C Mobility
0 = bed or chair bound
1 = able to get out of bed / chair but does not go out
2 = goes out ☐

D Has suffered psychological stress or acute disease in the past 3 months?
0 = yes   2 = no ☐

E Neuropsychological problems
0 = severe dementia or depression
1 = mild dementia
2 = no psychological problems ☐

F Body Mass Index (BMI) (weight in kg) / (height in m²)
0 = BMI less than 19
1 = BMI 19 to less than 21
2 = BMI 21 to less than 23
3 = BMI 23 or greater ☐

Screening score (subtotal max. 14 points) ☐☐
12-14 points: Normal nutritional status
8-11 points: At risk of malnutrition
0-7 points: Malnourished
For a more in-depth assessment, continue with questions G-R

Assessment

G Lives independently (not in nursing home or hospital)
1 = yes   0 = no ☐

H Takes more than 3 prescription drugs per day
0 = yes   1 = no ☐

I Pressure sores or skin ulcers
0 = yes   1 = no ☐

J How many full meals does the patient eat daily?
0 = 1 meal
1 = 2 meals
2 = 3 meals ☐

K Selected consumption markers for protein intake
- At least one serving of dairy products (milk, cheese, yoghurt) per day   yes ☐ no ☐
- Two or more servings of legumes or eggs per week   yes ☐ no ☐
- Meat, fish or poultry every day   yes ☐ no ☐
0.0 = if 0 or 1 yes
0.5 = if 2 yes
1.0 = if 3 yes ☐.☐

L Consumes two or more servings of fruit or vegetables per day?
0 = no   1 = yes ☐

M How much fluid (water, juice, coffee, tea, milk...) is consumed per day?
0.0 = less than 3 cups
0.5 = 3 to 5 cups
1.0 = more than 5 cups ☐.☐

N Mode of feeding
0 = unable to eat without assistance
1 = self-fed with some difficulty
2 = self-fed without any problem ☐

O Self view of nutritional status
0 = views self as being malnourished
1 = is uncertain of nutritional state
2 = views self as having no nutritional problem ☐

P In comparison with other people of the same age, how does the patient consider his / her health status?
0.0 = not as good
0.5 = does not know
1.0 = as good
2.0 = better ☐.☐

Q Mid-arm circumference (MAC) in cm
0.0 = MAC less than 21
0.5 = MAC 21 to 22
1.0 = MAC greater than 22 ☐.☐

R Calf circumference (CC) in cm
0 = CC less than 31
1 = CC 31 or greater ☐

Assessment (max. 16 points) ☐☐.☐
Screening score ☐☐.☐
Total Assessment (max. 30 points) ☐☐.☐

Malnutrition Indicator Score
24 to 30 points	☐	Normal nutritional status
17 to 23.5 points	☐	At risk of malnutrition
Less than 17 points	☐	Malnourished

References
1. Vellas B, Villars H, Abellan G, *et al.* Overview of the MNA® - Its History and Challenges. *J Nutr Health Aging.* 2006; **10:456**-465.
2. Rubenstein LZ, Harker JO, Salva A, Guigoz Y, Vellas B. Screening for Undernutrition in Geriatric Practice: Developing the Short-Form Mini Nutritional Assessment (MNA-SF). *J. Geront.* 2001; **56A**: M366-377
3. Guigoz Y. The Mini-Nutritional Assessment (MNA®) Review of the Literature - What does it tell us? *J Nutr Health Aging.* 2006; **10**:466-487.
® Société des Produits Nestlé, S.A., Vevey, Switzerland, Trademark Owners
© Nestlé, 1994, Revision 2009. N67200 12/99 10M
For more information: www.mna-elderly.com

NCLEX®-STYLE REVIEW QUESTIONS

Read each question carefully. Choose the best answer for each question.

1. The nurse is aware that undernutrition may lead to:
   1. muscle loss
   2. a compromised immune system
   3. poor wound healing
   4. All of the above

2. When using a diet recall as part of a nutritional assessment, it is best for the nurse to:
   1. encourage the client to record his intake for one full week
   2. encourage the client to record his intake for a weekday and a weekend day
   3. encourage the client to record his intake for five weekdays and two full weekends
   4. encourage the client to record his intake for 30 days

3. The nurse understands that anthropometric measurements refer to:
   1. height, weight, body mass index, and abdominal circumference
   2. the overall increase in the average size of humans throughout history
   3. the tracking of an individual's measurements from infancy through late adulthood
   4. the use of the metric system when measuring height and weight ratios

4. A 62-year-old male reports to the clinic for his annual physical assessment. His present weight is 174 lb, and his last recorded weight was 198 lb four months ago. He claims he has had a very poor appetite for the past few months, and he denies doing any exercise. The nurse interprets this finding as a weight loss:
   1. of 2% and of no clinical significance
   2. of 8% and of clinical significance
   3. greater than 11% and of clinical significance
   4. greater than 15% and of no clinical significance

5. The equipment needed for the nurse to obtain skinfold thickness measurements includes:
   1. calipers
   2. calipers and a flexible measuring tape
   3. a flexible measuring tape and 5-lb dumbbell
   4. calipers, flexible measuring tape, and a 5-lb dumbbell

6. A 16-year-old girl is on the cheerleading squad at her high school. She has just completed her sports health clearance assessment. The nurse would be concerned with which findings? (Select all that apply.)
   1. A BMI that dropped from the 25th percentile to the 5th percentile
   2. Restricting her calories to 1800 to 2000 calories per day
   3. Consumes three to four energy drinks daily
   4. Avoids all carbohydrates and meats in order to lose weight quickly
   5. Runs 3 miles per day to stay fit for the squad

7. A young adult is admitted through the emergency department for alcohol intoxication. The client has a long history of alcohol abuse. To complete a comprehensive initial assessment, the nurse anticipates which lab tests to be ordered in order to evaluate visceral protein status?
   1. Nitrogen and cholesterol
   2. Albumin and prealbumin
   3. Nitrogen and albumin
   4. Cholesterol and triglycerides

8. The nurse is aware that the culture of a client may influence the: (Select all that apply.)
   1. method of food preparation
   2. number of meals eaten in a day
   3. types of herbs used
   4. food selection for special occasions
   5. food beliefs

9. An 81-year-old male was brought to the emergency department due to a syncopal episode (fainting). A 12-lead EKG has revealed that the patient has an arrhythmia called *torsades de pointes*. This arrhythmia is commonly caused by:
   1. a magnesium deficiency
   2. a sodium deficiency
   3. an iron deficiency
   4. a vitamin D deficiency

10. When performing a nutritional assessment, it is important for the nurse to collect data regarding a client's functional capacity because the client may not be capable of: (Select all that apply.)
    1. food shopping
    2. feeding himself
    3. preparing a meal
    4. reading a food label
    5. opening containers when preparing a meal

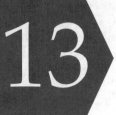

13 > Skin, Hair, and Nails

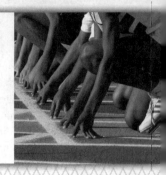

All the world is a laboratory to the inquiring mind.
—Martin H. Fischer

The integumentary system includes the skin, hair, and nails. It can reveal vital information about multiple systems when thoroughly and accurately assessed. This chapter will focus on gathering both subjective and objective data and on analysis of the data collected.

OBJECTIVES

At the completion of these exercises, you will be able to:

1. Review the anatomy and physiology of the integumentary system.
2. Apply lifespan considerations related to assessment of the integumentary system.
3. Identify the correct techniques for assessment of the integumentary system.
4. Analyze subjective and objective data related to assessment of the integumentary system.
5. Recognize factors that can influence assessment findings.
6. Apply critical thinking in analysis of a case study.
7. Assess the integumentary system on a laboratory partner.
8. Document an assessment of the integumentary system.
9. Complete NCLEX®-style review questions related to assessment of the integumentary system.

ANATOMY & PHYSIOLOGY REVIEW

For each diagram below, label the structures as indicated by each line.

1.

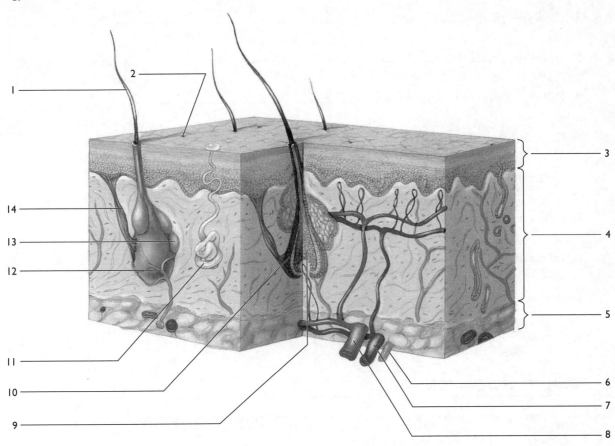

2.

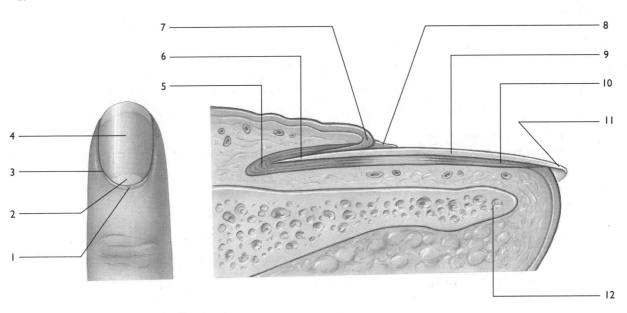

3. Read each statement. On the line provided indicate if the characteristic is a function of the skin, subcutaneous gland, or neither.

   1. Perceives pain _____

   2. Creates perspiration _____

   3. Synthesizes vitamin D _____

   4. Protects against environmental toxins _____

   5. Creates mucus _____

   6. Protects against bacterial growth _____

   7. Excretes vitamin D _____

   8. Lubricates _____

   9. Perceives touch _____

   10. Converts vitamin C into uric acid _____

LIFESPAN CONSIDERATIONS

Review each statement and write the rationale for the age-related consideration on the line provided.

1. As adults age, they begin to develop wrinkles on the skin.

   Rationale: _____

2. It is not advisable to apply topical medications to the skin of infants under 6 months of age.

   Rationale: _____

3. As adults age, their hair color changes to grayish white.

   Rationale: _____

4. Infants are at a greater risk of heat intolerance than young adults.

   Rationale: _____

ASSESSMENT TECHNIQUES

Review each assessment technique. If the technique is correct, circle the number. If the technique is incorrect, write the correct assessment technique on the line provided.

1. When examining a client's skin, it is best to have the client fully disrobed and in a supine position on an examination table.

   _____

   _____

2. Explain that you will be touching the client in various areas with different parts of your hand.

   _____

   _____

3. It is best to determine a client's skin temperature using the ulnar surface of the hand.

    _____

    _____

4. When palpating for skin texture, it is best to use the palmar surface of the fingers and finger pads.

    _____

    _____

5. Skin turgor can be assessed on the adult by using the forefinger and thumb to grasp the skin superior to the clavicle or on the lateral aspect of the wrist.

    _____

    _____

6. The assessment technique used to grade edema on a four-point scale is inspection.

    _____

    _____

7. When assessing a client's scalp and hair, it is best to divide the hair at 1-inch intervals.

    _____

    _____

8. When assessing for hair texture, it is appropriate to roll a few strands of hair between your thumb and forefinger.

    _____

    _____

9. Capillary refill can be assessed by depressing the cuticle briefly to blanch and then quickly releasing.

    _____

    _____

10. The spooning technique can be performed to assess clubbing.

    _____

    _____

ASSESSMENT FINDINGS

Read each assessment finding. Determine if the finding is normal or abnormal by writing an "N" for normal or an "A" for abnormal on each line provided.

_____ **1.** Pallor		_____ **11.** +2 edema	
_____ **2.** Warm and dry		_____ **12.** Ecchymoses	
_____ **3.** Jaundice		_____ **13.** Tinea capitis	
_____ **4.** Free from odor		_____ **14.** Thick hair	
_____ **5.** Freckles		_____ **15.** Brittle hair	
_____ **6.** Fine network of thin veins on the eyelids		_____ **16.** Bluish tint to nail beds	
_____ **7.** Fine sheen of perspiration		_____ **17.** Gray scaly patches on scalp	
_____ **8.** Smooth and firm		_____ **18.** 160° nail curvature	
_____ **9.** Pruritus		_____ **19.** Spoon nails	
_____ **10.** Decreased skin turgor		_____ **20.** Senile lentigines	

FACTORS THAT INFLUENCE PHYSICAL ASSESSMENT FINDINGS

Fill in the blank(s) to complete each statement.

1. When assessing dark-skinned clients for skin color changes, it is best to inspect the _____, _____, _____, and _____.

2. The fine, downy hair on a newborn is replaced with _____ hair within a few months.

3. The older adult has a/an _____ in sweat gland activity.

4. Many _____ females develop striae gravidarum.

5. Adolescents are prone to _____ because of the increased production of sebum.

6. Compulsive behaviors related to stress may be demonstrated by _____ or _____.

ABNORMAL FINDINGS

Write the name of each lesion on the first line next to each illustration. On the second line write two associated characteristics. Finally, on the third line provide an example of that type of lesion.

Example

Cyst

Fluid filled and elevated

Sebaceous cysts

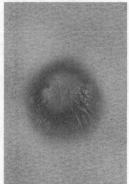

1. _____

_____

_____

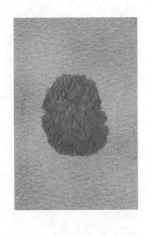

2. _____
_____
_____

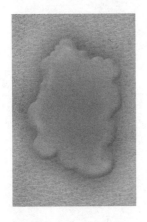

3. _____
_____
_____

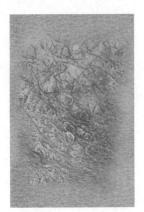

4. _____
_____
_____

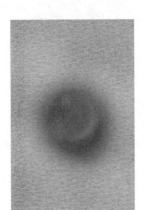

5. _____
_____
_____

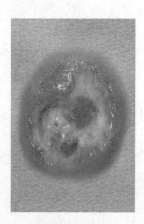

6. _____
   _____
   _____

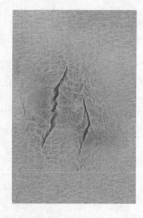

7. _____
   _____
   _____

8. _____
   _____
   _____

APPLICATION OF THE CRITICAL THINKING PROCESS

Read each of the scenarios below and then answer the questions that follow in the space provided.

SCENARIO A

Mr. Young is a 22-year-old male who presents to a clinic with symptoms of a common cold. After gathering data for a health history, you learn that he has worked for his father's landscape company since he was 16 years old. When assessing his posterior thorax for breath sounds, you notice a 5-mm × 2-mm lesion on the posterior neck. When you question Mr. Young about this lesion, he states "I could feel something there but I thought it was a patch of dry skin." He also states that it has been there for at least 6 months. You learn that Mr. Young does not apply sunscreen to his body when he is landscaping and often removes his shirt when he feels too hot. As you continue to assess the lesion, you note it has rounded pearly edges with a central mild ulceration.

1. Identify two subjective behaviors presented by Mr. Young.

    A.

    B.

2. Identify two objective behaviors noted by the nurse.

    A.

    B.

3. List two risk factors identified by Mr. Young.

    A.

    B.

4. What type of lesion do you suspect this to be?

During the remainder of the assessment, you learn that Mr. Young intermittently experiences a stinging sensation at the site of the lesion. He began experiencing this when he first noticed the lesion 6 months ago.

5. Place the data collected into the OLDCART & ICE assessment. If the assessment is incomplete, write questions that the nurse should ask to complete the assessment.

    O

    L

D

C

A

R

T

I

C

E

6. Explain the ABCDE criteria for skin cancer screening.

A

B

C

D

E

7. Consider the *Healthy People 2020* objective "Reduce the rate of sunburn." Explain how a nurse could have used this objective to prevent skin cancer in Mr. Young.

SCENARIO B

Julia is a 6-year-old girl who was sent to the school nurse's office for an itch on her scalp. She states it started the night before and is becoming very annoying. After putting on a pair of clean gloves, you begin to inspect her long, light blonde hair and note tiny white nits along multiple hair shafts. You also note her scalp in the occipital region is reddened and excoriated. You determine that Julia has pediculosis capitis. (Additional resources may be necessary to complete this scenario.)

1. List the subjective and objective data gathered that led you to this conclusion.

   Subjective data:

   Objective data:

2. Can Julia be sent back to class? Explain.

3. What teaching must be done and with whom in this situation?

4. State your learning goal for the client and/or parent.

5. Write two objectives to support your learning goal from Question 4.

   A.

   B.

6. Explain how you will evaluate the goal stated in Question 4.

ASSESSMENT AND DOCUMENTATION

Perform an integumentary assessment on your lab partner and document your findings on the following documentation form.

SKIN, HAIR, AND NAILS

Name:_____Date:_____

Age: _____ Gender: _____

FOCUSED INTERVIEW

Reason for today's visit:_____

_____

General Questions

Describe your skin today: _____

Describe any changes in your skin in the past:

    2 weeks: _____

    2 months: _____

    2 years: _____

Describe your hair today: _____

    Describe any recent changes: _____

Describe your nails today: _____

    Describe any recent changes: _____

Allergies: _____

Recent illness: _____

Current medical conditions: _____

Prescription or over-the-counter medication: _____

Describe your diet: _____

Describe any disorders you have related to:

    Skin: _____

    Hair: _____

    Nails: _____

Describe any disorders your family members have related to:

    Skin: _____

    Hair: _____

    Nails: _____

Hygiene practices:

    Skin: _____

    Hair: _____

    Nails: _____

Sun exposure:

    Natural: _____

    Artificial: _____

    Protection: _____

Occupational/chemical exposures: _____

Recent travel (if yes, where?): _____

Skin: Symptoms or Behaviors

Do you now or have you ever had:

    Sores/ulcerations: _____

    Itching: _____

Prolonged emotional upset or anxiety: _____

Rash: _____

Moles: _____

Birthmarks: _____

Tattoo(s): _____

Sunburn: _____

Piercings: _____

Lesions: _____

Scars: _____

Color changes: _____

Changes in sweating: _____

Oily or dry skin: _____

Odor: _____

Pain/discomfort:

    O
    L
    D
    C
    A
    R
    T
    I
    C
    E

Hair: Symptoms or Behaviors

Do you now or have you ever had:

Hair loss:

    Head: _____

    Body: _____

Pattern: _____

Excessive hair growth: _____

Hair removal: _____

Color changes: _____

Flaking/dandruff: _____

Nails: Symptoms or Behaviors

Do you now or have you ever had:

Nail biting: _____

Splitting/peeling: _____

Ridges/grooves: _____

Redness/swelling to cuticles: _____

Color changes: _____

Artificial nails/tips/wraps: _____

Pain/discomfort: _____

Age-Related Questions

Infants and Children

Any birthmarks? If so, where are they?

Developed an orange hue to the skin?

Rash? If so, what seems to have caused it?

Any burns, bruises, scrapes, or other injuries?

Menstruating Females

Are you pregnant? If not, are you menstruating regularly? Describe your menstrual periods.

Pregnant Females

Noticed any changes in your skin since you became pregnant?

Do you use any topical medication for problems with the skin, hair, or nails?

Do you use topical medications for other problems? If so, list the medications.

Older Adults

What changes have you noticed in your skin in the past few years?

Does your skin itch?

Do you experience frequent falls?

PHYSICAL ASSESSMENT

Skin

Inspection

Cleanliness: _____

Odor: _____

Tone: _____

Pigmentation: _____

Superficial arteries/veins: _____

Lesions: _____

Location: Place a mark on the following body outline to represent lesions found on the skin of the client. Number the lesions.

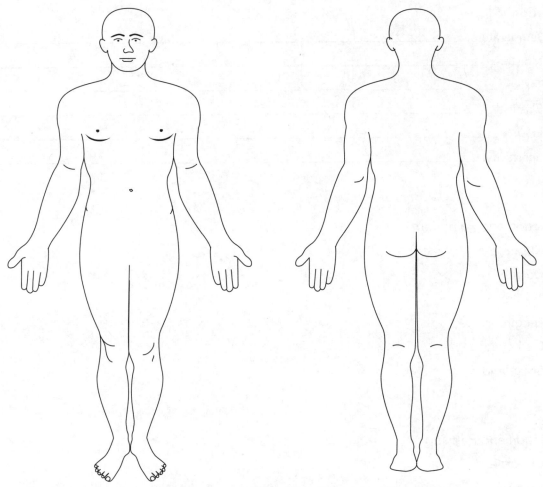

Source: Copyright Colleen Barbarito and Donita D'Amico.

Complete an in-depth assessment of three lesions using the assigned numbers from the above body outline.

	Lesion 1	**Lesion 2**	**Lesion 3**
Configuration:			
Size:			
Shape:			
Drainage:			
Color:			
Odor:			
Consistency:			
Amount:			
Location:			
Cancer Screening:			
A:			
B:			
C:			
D:			
E:			

Palpation

Temperature: _____

Moisture: _____

Texture: _____

Elasticity: _____

Edema: _____

Sensitivity: _____

Hair

Inspection and Palpation

Cleanliness:

Color:

Texture:

Length:

Distribution:

Scalp lesions:

Nails

Inspection and Palpation

Cleanliness:

Color:

Capillary refill:

Shape/contour:

Schamroth technique:

Cuticles:

Comments:

NCLEX®-STYLE REVIEW QUESTIONS

Read each question carefully. Choose the best answer for each question.

1. The nurse knows that which of the following are major functions of the skin? (Select all that apply.)
   1. Perception of pain and pressure
   2. Regulation of body temperature
   3. Vitamin E synthesis
   4. Protection from ultraviolet rays
   5. Protection against bacterial invasion

2. The nurse knows that which of the following are considered vascular lesions? (Select all that apply.)
   1. Port-wine stain
   2. Hematoma
   3. Petechia
   4. Keloid
   5. Pustule

3. The nurse is aware that the older adult may experience which of the following changes in the integumentary system?
    1. Decrease in the number of sweat glands
    2. Increase in skin elasticity
    3. Increased coarse facial hair
    4. Decreased sebum production

4. A client is asking a nurse questions about skin cancer. The nurse explains to the client that the least common but most serious type of skin cancer is:
    1. basal cell carcinoma
    2. squamous cell carcinoma
    3. malignant melanoma
    4. Kaposi's sarcoma

5. A nurse is assessing the nails of a newly admitted client to a long-term care facility. She notes redness, swelling, and tenderness to the cuticle of the third and fourth left digits. This is also known as:
    1. hirsutism
    2. paronychia
    3. onycholysis
    4. folliculitis

6. When assessing a client's nails, the nurse notices horizontal white bands in multiple fingers. This could indicate:
    1. arteriosclerosis
    2. hepatic or renal disease
    3. hypoxia
    4. vitamin deficiencies

7. Skin turgor assesses the elasticity and mobility of the skin. The nurse knows that which of the following is true about skin turgor? Skin turgor is: (Select all that apply.)
    1. decreased in dehydrated clients
    2. decreased in clients with scleroderma
    3. decreased in clients who have lost large amounts of weight
    4. increased in clients with connective tissue disorders that harden the skin
    5. increased turgor that results in tenting of the skin

8. Which of the following lesions would the nurse consider abnormal when assessing the skin of an older adult client?
    1. Cherry angiomas
    2. Cutaneous tags
    3. Senile lentigines
    4. Chloasma

9. A nurse working in the emergency department is assessing a rectal temperature on an Asian newborn. The nurse notices a bluish-purple discoloration to the sacral area. The nurse's next step should be to:
    1. notify the Division of Youth and Family Services for suspected abuse
    2. bring the child to the attention of the healthcare provider immediately because of suspected trauma
    3. continue with her assessment and disregard the finding
    4. seek clarification with the parents that the discoloration is a Mongolian spot

10. Spoon nails are commonly associated with:
    1. iron deficiency
    2. vitamin B_1 deficiency
    3. vitamin D deficiency
    4. deficiency of fat-soluble vitamins

 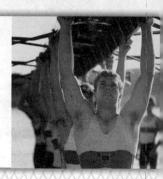

14 · Head, Neck, and Related Lymphatics

The will to win is important, but the will to prepare is vital.
—Joe Paterno

The head and neck may appear to be a small region in relation to the rest of the body; however, a thorough assessment of this region can lead to vital information in other body systems. This chapter will focus on gathering both subjective and objective data, as well as analysis of the data collected.

OBJECTIVES

At the completion of these exercises, you will be able to:

1. Review the anatomy and physiology of the head, neck, and related lymphatics.
2. Identify the correct techniques for assessment of the head, neck, and related lymphatics.
3. Analyze subjective and objective data related to assessment of the head, neck, and related lymphatics.
4. Recognize factors that can influence assessment findings.
5. Apply critical thinking in analysis of a case study.
6. Relate *Healthy People 2020* objectives to the head, neck, and related lymphatics.
7. Assess the head, neck, and related lymphatics on a laboratory partner.
8. Document an assessment of the head, neck, and related lymphatics.
9. Complete NCLEX®-style review questions related to assessment of the head, neck, and related lymphatics.

ANATOMY & PHYSIOLOGY REVIEW

1. For each of the following diagrams, label the structures as indicated by each line.

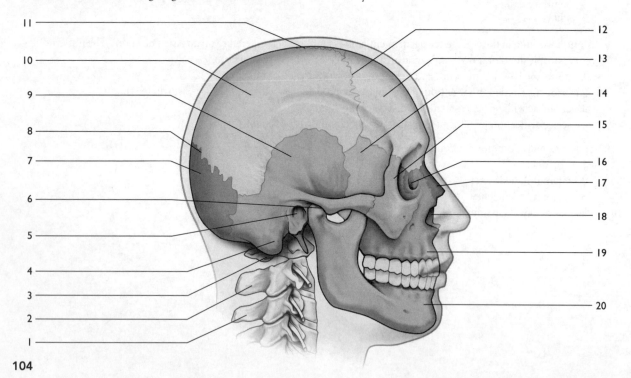

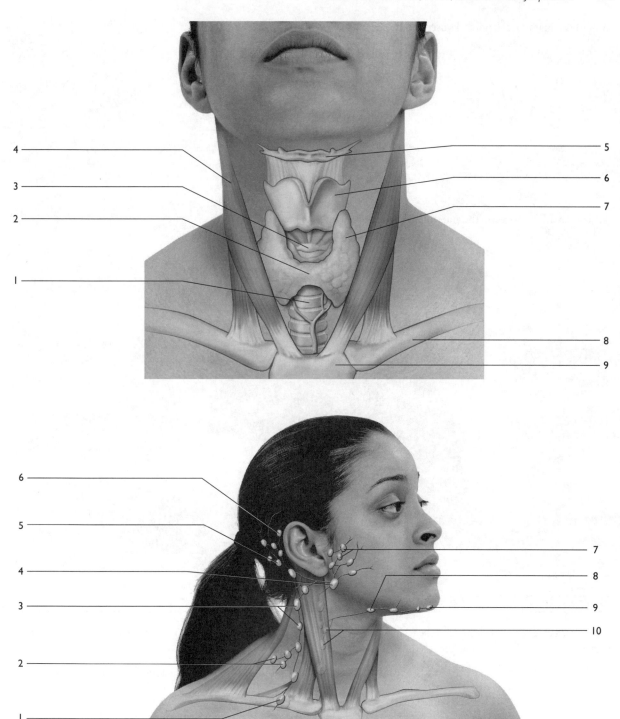

2. List the anatomical landmarks used for the anterior triangle of the neck:

   1.

   2.

   3.

3. List the anatomical landmarks used for the posterior triangle of the neck:

   1.

   2.

   3.

4. Use a pencil to shade in the anterior and posterior triangles of the neck.

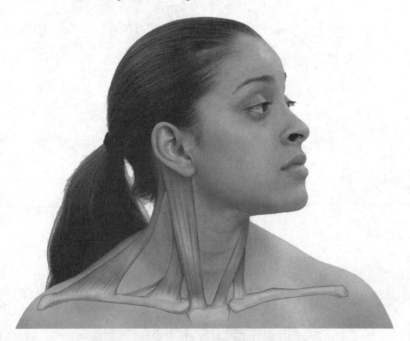

ASSESSMENT TECHNIQUES

Review each assessment technique. If the technique is correct, circle the number. If the technique is incorrect, write the correct assessment technique on the line provided.

1. When examining a client's head and neck, it is best to have the client fully disrobed and in a supine position on an examination table.

_____

_____

2. Explain that you will be touching the client in various areas with different parts of your hand.

_____

_____

3. Explain to the client the need to remove items that would interfere with the assessment, such as hair clips, hats, scarves, veils, or jewelry.

_____

_____

4. Palpate for the temporal artery between the trachea and sternocleidomastoid using the finger pads.

_____

_____

5. When palpating the thyroid gland by standing behind the client, the examiner's left hand will push the trachea to the right. The thyroid would be palpated with the examiner's right hand.

_____

_____

6. The thyroid cannot be auscultated for bruits.

_____

_____

7. Lymph nodes are palpated by exerting moderate pressure in a vertical motion.

_____

_____

8. The best order to examine the lymph nodes of the head and neck is from the cervical chains to the jaw followed by the supraclavicular region.

_____

_____

9. The trachea should be palpated using the thumb and the index finger.

_____

_____

10. Percussion of the trachea is best done with a bimanual method.

_____

_____

ASSESSMENT FINDINGS

Read each assessment finding. Identify the finding as normal or abnormal by writing an "N" for normal or an "A" for abnormal on each line provided.

_____ 1. Nasolabial folds equal

_____ 2. Facial movements smooth

_____ 3. TMJ crepitation

_____ 4. Nuchal rigidity

_____ 5. Smooth trachea

_____ 6. Nonpalpable thyroid in newborns

_____ 7. Lymphadenopathy

_____ 8. Tenderness to the temporal artery

_____ 9. Jugular vein distention

_____ 10. Movement of the trachea when client swallows

_____ 11. Scaliness of the scalp

_____ 12. Normocephalic

_____ 13. Unilateral facial paralysis

_____ 14. Slight tremors of the lips

_____ 15. Torticollis

_____ 16. Hyperextension of the neck

_____ 17. Goiter

_____ 18. Thyroid bruit

_____ 19. Nonpalpable occipital node

_____ 20. Tenderness to scalp

FACTORS THAT INFLUENCE PHYSICAL ASSESSMENT FINDINGS

Fill in the blank to complete each statement.

1. Thyroid disorders are common in areas where _____ is limited.

2. The ability for an infant to control his or her head occurs at about _____ months.

3. The older female adult may develop coarse hair on the _____.

4. A disorder that may be seen in infants whose mothers ingest significant amounts of alcohol during pregnancy is called _____ _____ _____.

5. The posterior fontanel is a/an _____.

6. The _____ adult loses subcutaneous fat in the face.

7. Psychological stress may lead to physical pain, most commonly in the _____ or _____.

8. The thyroid may _____ in size during pregnancy.

9. In the Muslim culture it is common for the females to cover their _____ and _____.

10. The range of motion (ROM) of the cervical spine may be limited because of _____ of the vertebrae.

APPLICATION OF THE CRITICAL THINKING PROCESS

Read the scenario below and then answer the questions that follow in the space provided.

Ronnie is a 22-year-old African American male who works for the environmental services department at a small community hospital. He cleans client rooms upon discharge and maintains the cleanliness of the hallways. Everyone at the hospital knows Ronnie because he is always friendly and always smiling. Over the past 2 months, Ronnie hasn't been his usual cheerful self and has appeared very sweaty and anxious at times while performing his typical duties. When asked if anything is wrong, he simply states "I haven't been sleeping well at night." He also apprehensively reveals that his stomach "hasn't been right" and that he has been having "frequent episodes of diarrhea." His face appears thinner, and he admits to losing 12 lb in the past month or so.

1. List five pieces of subjective data in the above scenario:

    1.

    2.

    3.

    4.

    5.

Ronnie is seen in the emergency department the next day, when he complains of heart palpitations and a slight uncontrollable tremor in his left hand.

2. List five questions the nurse should ask Ronnie on his arrival at the emergency department.

   1.

   2.

   3.

   4.

   5.

During the health history, the nurse notices that Ronnie has exophthalmus. When further investigating this finding, Ronnie states he seldom looks at himself in a mirror and has not noticed the bulging of his eyes. He states that he thinks he may need a stronger eyeglasses prescription because his vision has been more blurry than usual.

3. Define exophthalmus.

4. What may be responsible for Ronnie's variety of signs and symptoms?

5. Write three focused interview questions that would assist in gathering further data from Ronnie.

   1.

   2.

   3.

6. Use OLDCART & ICE to identify data related to pain.

7. List the questions the nurse should ask to complete the pain assessment.

HEALTHY PEOPLE 2020

Read the Healthy People 2020 *objective and answer the questions that follow in the space provided.*
A Healthy People 2020 *objective is:*

Increase the proportion of motorcyclists using helmets.

1. What are the laws in your city or town related to helmet use for cyclists? Is this a local or state ordinance?

2. Discuss how a nurse can use this objective to promote and maintain the health and optimal function of the structures of the head and neck.

ASSESSMENT AND DOCUMENTATION

Perform a head, neck, and lymphatic assessment on your lab partner and document your findings on the following documentation form.

HEAD, NECK, AND RELATED LYMPHATICS

Name:_____Date:_____

Age: _____ Gender: _____

FOCUSED INTERVIEW

Reason for today's visit: _____

_____

General Questions

Describe the condition of your head and neck today: _____

Describe any changes in your head and neck in the past:

    2 weeks: _____

    2 months: _____

    2 years: _____

Allergies: _____

Recent illness: _____

Current medical conditions: _____

Current medications (prescribed, over the counter, and herbal or home therapies): _____

Describe any disorders you have related to:

    Head: _____

    Face: _____

    Neck: _____

Thyroid gland: _____

Lymphatic system: _____

Describe any disorders your family members have related to:

Head: _____

Face: _____

Neck: _____

Thyroid gland: _____

Lymphatic system: _____

Describe any recent or past injury to your head: _____

Did you become unconscious? _____

Do you have headaches? _____

Frequency: _____

Onset: _____

Location: _____

Duration: _____

Character: _____

Associated symptoms: _____

Radiation: _____

Treatments: _____

Precipitating factors: _____

Symptoms or Behaviors

Do you now or have you ever had:

Dizziness: _____

Loss of consciousness: _____

Seizures: _____

Blurred vision: _____

Pain/discomfort: _____

Swelling, lumps, bumps, or sores on head or neck: _____

Alcohol, recreational drug, tobacco, or caffeine use:_____

O

L

D

C

A

R

T

I

C

E

Age-Related Questions

Infants and Children

Alcohol or drug use during pregnancy:_____

Depression or bulging over infant's "soft spots":_____

Pregnant Females

Frequent headaches: _____

Changes in skin on face:_____

Thyroid disease: _____

Older Adults

Safety precautions in the home: _____

Safety precautions outside of home (seat belt, assistive device use, etc.): _____

Environment

Stress, anxiety, or emotional upset: _____

History of head or neck irradiation: _____

Exposure to chemical toxins in the home or at work:_____

PHYSICAL ASSESSMENT

Head

Inspection

    Size: _____

    Shape: _____

    Symmetry: _____

    Integrity: _____

Palpation

    Temporal artery: _____

Auscultation

    Temporal artery: _____

Scalp/Hair

Inspection

    Hair distribution: _____

    Hair loss: _____

    Color: _____

    Hygiene: _____

    Itching/flaking of scalp: _____

    Lesions: _____

    Integrity: _____

Palpation

    Texture: _____

    Lumps/nodules: _____

Face

Inspection

Facial expressions: _____

Symmetry of structures

Eyes: _____

Brows: _____

Lashes: _____

Lids: _____

Ears: _____

Lips: _____

Nasolabial folds: _____

Palpebral fissures: _____

Brows to pupils: Right: _____   Left: _____

Outer canthus to pinna: Right: _____   Left: _____

Movements: _____

TMJ:

ROM: _____

Symmetry of movement: _____

Lesions: _____

Swelling: _____

Weakness: _____

Palpation

TMJ: Right: _____   Left: _____

Temporal artery: Right: _____   Left: _____

Neck

Inspection

Skin color: _____

Integrity: _____

Symmetry: _____

ROM: _____

Carotid arteries: Right: _____   Left: _____

Jugular veins: Internal: Right: _____   Left: _____

   External: Right: _____   Left: _____

Trachea: _____

Thyroid gland: _____

Palpation

Carotid arteries: Right: _____   Left: _____

Trachea: _____

Thyroid gland: _____

Auscultation

Carotid arteries: Right: _____   Left: _____

Thyroid gland: _____

Lymph Nodes

	Palpable		Comments
Preauricular	_____No	_____Yes	_____
Postauricular	_____No	_____Yes	_____
Occipital	_____No	_____Yes	_____
Retropharyngeal	_____No	_____Yes	_____
Submandibular	_____No	_____Yes	_____
Submental	_____No	_____Yes	_____
Superficial cervical chain	_____No	_____Yes	_____
Deep cervical chain	_____No	_____Yes	_____
Supraclavicular	_____No	_____Yes	_____

Comments: _____

_____

_____

NCLEX®-STYLE REVIEW QUESTIONS

Read each question carefully. Choose the best answer for each question.

1. The nurse knows that mobility in the cervical spine is greatest at the level of:
    1. C_1, C_2, and C_3
    2. C_3, C_4, and C_5
    3. C_4, C_5, and C_6
    4. C_5, C_6, and C_7

2. The nurse understands that the anterior fontanelle is formed by:
    1. the coronal suture, frontal suture, and sagittal suture
    2. the sagittal suture, lambdoidal suture, and coronal suture
    3. the coronal suture, frontal suture, and lambdoidal suture
    4. the sagittal suture, frontal suture, and lambdoidal suture

3. Which of the following questions would be **inappropriate** for the nurse to ask when conducting a focused interview with a client who has suffered an acute head injury?
    1. "Did anyone witness your injury?"
    2. "Have you experienced nausea or vomiting since your injury?"
    3. "Where on your head are you experiencing pain?"
    4. "How often do you wash your hair?"

4. The nurse knows that enlarged palpable lymph nodes may be indicative of:
    1. malignancy or infection
    2. infection or thrombosis
    3. vascular occlusion or malignancy
    4. thrombosis or vascular occlusion

5. An infant is diagnosed with fetal alcohol syndrome. The nurse performs an assessment and knows that which of the following assessment findings supports this diagnosis?
    1. Deformed upper lip
    2. Widened palpebral fissures
    3. Deep nasolabial folds
    4. "Moon" face

6. The nurse understands an increased production of growth hormone can lead to:
    1. hydrocephalus
    2. craniosynostosis
    3. Cushing's syndrome
    4. acromegaly

7. A client presents to a busy urban emergency department complaining of pain that radiates from the base of the cervical spine to the right frontal region of the head. The client describes the pain as a dull, steady ache that began in the morning and has gradually increased in intensity throughout the day. The nurse identifies these symptoms most likely indicate a:
    1. cluster headache
    2. tension headache
    3. spinal headache
    4. classic migraine

8. The nurse is examining a client's neck. Which of the following movements of the neck will the nurse assess when testing range of motion (ROM)? (Select all that apply.)
    1. Turn head to right and left
    2. Rotate head in a circular fashion
    3. Extend head back
    4. Stick out tongue
    5. Tuck chin to chest

9. An adult client presents to the outpatient clinic with a 2-day history of shortness of breath. While at the clinic, the client's respiratory rate increases rapidly, and the client appears cyanotic. The nurse notes the client's trachea is deviated from the midline. The nurse identifies that this client is most likely experiencing:
    1. pneumothorax
    2. lung cancer
    3. myocardial infarction
    4. pulmonary embolism

10. The nurse is assessing a client's ear. The top of the ear should align directly with the:
    1. pinna
    2. nasolabial folds
    3. brow
    4. lateral canthus

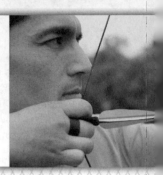

It is better to trust the eyes than the ears.
—German Proverb

The eye is a sensory organ that is responsible for vision. A thorough assessment of the eye will include structural, visual, and neuromuscular testing. This chapter will focus on gathering both subjective and objective data, as well as analysis of the data collected:

OBJECTIVES

At the completion of these exercises, you will be able to:

1. Review the anatomy and physiology of the eye.
2. Identify the correct techniques for assessment of the eye.
3. Analyze subjective and objective data related to assessment of the eye.
4. Recognize factors that can influence assessment findings.
5. Apply critical thinking in analysis of a case study.
6. Relate *Healthy People 2020* objectives to the eye.
7. Perform an assessment of the eye on your laboratory partner.
8. Document an assessment of the eye.
9. Complete NCLEX®-style review questions related to the assessment of the eye.

ANATOMY & PHYSIOLOGY REVIEW

1. For each of the following diagrams, label the structures as indicated by each line.

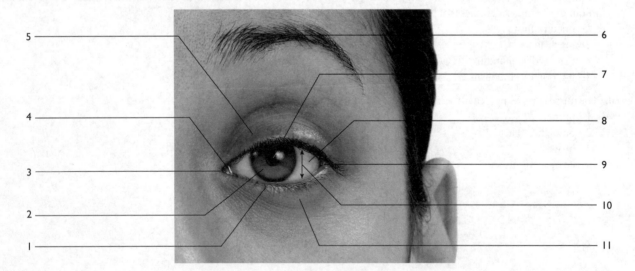

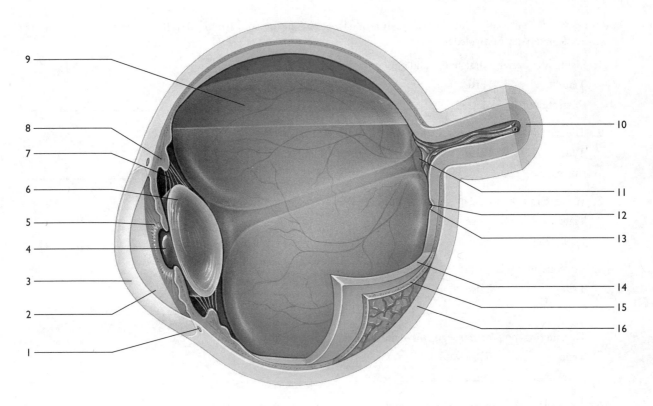

9
8
7
6
5
4
3
2
1

10
11
12
13
14
15
16

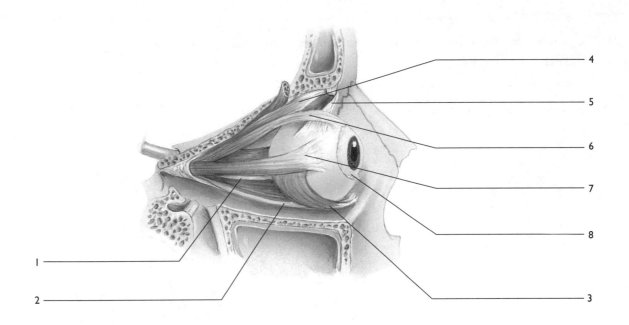

4
5
6
7
8

1
2
3

2. Read each statement carefully. Identify each as true or false by circling the word True or False. If the statement is false, rewrite it correctly in the space provided.

1. Light rays travel in a straight line and must refract in order for vision to occur.

True   **False**

Correction: _____

2. The crystalline lens is solely responsible for the refraction of light rays.

True   **False**

Correction: _____

3. When refraction occurs, the rays are reflected to the cornea for the most accurate vision.

True   **False**

Correction: _____

4. Aqueous humor is a refractory medium.

True   **False**

Correction: _____

5. The anterior and posterior segments of the eye are separated by the retina.

True   **False**

Correction: _____

6. A retinal image is conducted to the occipital nerve.

True   **False**

Correction: _____

7. The optic chiasm is the site for crossover of the nerve fingers.

True   **False**

Correction: _____

8. Impulses from the eye are transmitted to the temporal lobe of the brain for interpretation.

True   **False**

Correction: _____

3. Label each picture with the cranial nerves responsible for the eye movement.

1 _____

2 _____

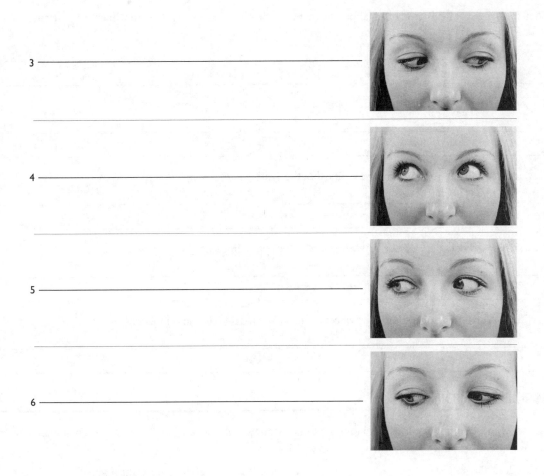

3 _____

4 _____

5 _____

6 _____

ASSESSMENT TECHNIQUES

Review each assessment technique. If the technique is correct, circle the number. If the technique is incorrect, write the correct assessment technique on the line provided.

1. Position the client approximately 40 inches away from the Rosenbaum chart to assess near vision.

   _____

   _____

2. When assessing distant vision with the Snellen chart, ask the client to remove eyeglasses first and then repeat with eyeglasses on.

   _____

   _____

3. When positioning a client to test the six cardinal fields of gaze, the nurse should be at eye level with the client.

   _____

   _____

4. To assess the corneal light reflex, the nurse should instruct the client to stare directly into the penlight.

   _____

   _____

5. When testing visual fields by confrontation, the client should be sitting about 1 foot from the nurse.

   _____

   _____

6. When testing visual fields by confrontation, the client should cover one eye with a card while the nurse covers his or her own opposite eye.

_____

_____

7. The corneal reflex is stimulated by gently wisping a piece of cotton on the cornea.

_____

_____

8. To evaluate pupillary response, the nurse should dim the lighting in the room.

_____

_____

9. To examine the client's right eye, the nurse should hold the ophthalmoscope in his or her left hand.

_____

_____

10. If a client's vision is hyperopic, the diopter wheel should be rotated into the plus numbers.

_____

_____

ASSESSMENT FINDINGS

Read each assessment finding. Identify the finding as normal or abnormal by writing an "N" for normal or an "A" for abnormal on each line provided.

_____ 1. 20/200 vision
_____ 2. Nystagmus
_____ 3. PERRLA
_____ 4. Bilateral blinking when one cornea is touched
_____ 5. Equal distance between palpebral fissures
_____ 6. Fine network of thin veins on the external eyelids
_____ 7. Red reflex of the pupil
_____ 8. Pink conjunctiva
_____ 9. Ptosis of the lids
_____ 10. Symmetrical reflection of light on the cornea

_____ 11. Dark spots on the retina
_____ 12. Emmetropia
_____ 13. Lack of convergence
_____ 14. Opaque lens
_____ 15. Irregular shape to the optic disc
_____ 16. Small white spot in the center of the macula
_____ 17. Firm eyeballs
_____ 18. Convergence
_____ 19. Presbyopia
_____ 20. Round and equal pupils

FACTORS THAT INFLUENCE PHYSICAL ASSESSMENT FINDINGS

Fill in the blank to complete each statement.

1. In the assessment of a 3-week-old baby girl with both parents of Irish descent, you expect the irises of her eyes to be _____ in color.

2. A female, 7 months pregnant, has been wearing her eyeglasses instead of her contacts for the past 2 weeks. This is most likely because pregnant women are prone to _____.

3. A 5-year-old visits the eye doctor for the first time. He learns that his eyes will be adult size when he is _____ years old.

4. A 52-year-old female, visiting a plastic surgeon, is complaining about a drooping appearance of her eyes. The surgeon explains to the client the drooping is caused by a loss of _____.

5. A 3-year-old from an underdeveloped area of Africa is experiencing blindness due to a deficiency of vitamin _____.

6. A 38-year-old female visits the tanning parlor three times per week. She also enjoys sunbathing as frequently as she can. She does not like to wear sunglasses or eye shields because she does not like the "tan lines." These practices will increase her risk for _____.

7. A general contractor who is responsible for building a science lab at the local junior college has learned it is important to wear _____ when he goes to work.

8. A 25-year-old female is being told by her ophthalmologist that she needs eyeglasses. He explains that her Hispanic culture has a/an _____ rate of visual impairments compared to other cultures.

9. An African American female has been diagnosed with diabetes. She is concerned because she has learned that uncontrolled diabetes can lead to diabetic retinopathy. This complication may lead to _____.

10. When the nurse is assessing the eyes of an Asian client, prominent _____ are noted.

APPLICATION OF THE CRITICAL THINKING PROCESS

Read the scenario below and then answer the questions that follow in the space provided.

Jordan is a 5-year-old girl in kindergarten. After recess she complains to her teacher that her right eye is bothering her. The teacher sends her to the school nurse, who looks at Jordan and believes she has pink eye (conjunctivitis).

1. What physical assessment findings would support the school nurse's assumption?

2. How will the nurse test Jordan's visual acuity? Explain your answer.

The school nurse continues to assess Jordan. The nurse plans to assess Jordan's pain level.

3. List two pain scales that would be appropriate for the nurse to use.

4. After Jordan is sent home with her mother, the school nurse visits the kindergarten class to review good hand hygiene practices with the students. Why would the nurse select this as a topic at this time?

HEALTHY PEOPLE 2020

Read the Healthy People 2020 *objective and answer the questions that follow in the space provided.*

A *Healthy People 2020* objective is:

Reduce the number of occupational eye injuries.

1. Name three occupations where eye safety should be a priority.

   1.

   2.

   3.

2. Discuss how an occupational health nurse can use this objective to promote and maintain the health and function of the structures of the eye.

ASSESSMENT AND DOCUMENTATION

Perform an eye assessment on your lab partner and document your findings on the following documentation form.

EYE

Name:_____Date:_____

Age: _____ Gender: _____

FOCUSED INTERVIEW

Reason for today's visit: _____

_____

General Questions

When was the date of your last eye exam? _____

What were the results of that exam? _____

Describe your vision today: _____

Describe any changes in your vision in the past:

    2 weeks: _____

    2 months: _____

    2 years: _____

Do you wear?

    Glasses: _____

    Contact lenses: _____

    Both: _____

    Reason for the above: _____

Allergies:_____

Recent illness: _____

Current medical conditions: _____

Current medications (prescription, over the counter, herbal or home remedies): _____

Describe any disorders you have related to the eyes:

    Disease: _____

    Infection: _____

    Injury:_____

    Foreign bodies:_____

    Surgery: _____

_____

Describe any disorders your family members have related to the eyes: _____

_____

How do you care for your eyes? _____

    Eye makeup/remover: _____

    Contact lens care: _____

    Sunglasses: _____

    Safety glasses: _____

    Chemical/irritant exposures: _____

Symptoms or Behaviors

Do you now or have you ever had:

    Blurred vision: _____

    Light sensitivity: _____

    Night vision: _____

    Floaters: _____

    Halos: _____

    Drainage/crusting: _____

    Redness: _____

    Pain/discomfort: _____

        O
        L
        D
        C
        A
        R
        T
        I
        C
        E

Age-Related Questions

Infants and Children

Mother have vaginal infection at delivery: _____

Eye ointment received after birth: _____

Preterm or full-term delivery: _____

Infant looks directly at provider? y/n Follows objects? y/n

Any concerns about child's eyesight?_____

Date of last vision examination: _____

Rubs eyes frequently?_____

Pregnant Females

Any changes in eyesight?_____

Older Adults

Dryness or burning of eyes? y/n _____

Difficulty seeing at night? _____

Bothered by bright lights? _____

Tested for glaucoma? _____

Date of last eye examination? _____

Environment

Family history of diabetes, hypertension, or glaucoma: _____

How many hours/day using computer: _____

Sports/hobbies: _____

PHYSICAL ASSESSMENT

Visual Acuity

Distance without correction _____ right eye   _____ left eye   _____ both eyes

Distance with correction _____ right eye   _____ left eye   _____ both eyes

Near without correction _____ inches from eyes

Near with correction _____ inches from eyes

Visual Fields

Positive all fields _____ yes   _____ no

Comments: _____

Six Cardinal Fields

Follows all fields _____ yes _____

Smooth muscle movement _____ yes _____

Nystagmus: _____

Method used: _____

Reflexes

Corneal light reflex: _____

Corneal reflex: _____

Fusion reflex (cover test): _____

Pupillary response: Right: _____ direct _____ consensual

   Left: _____ direct _____ consensual

Accommodation: _____

Convergence: _____

Eye Structures

Inspection

Eyebrows: _____

Eyelashes: _____

Eyelids: _____

Palpebral fissures: _____

Irises: _____

Pupils: _____

Conjunctiva: _____

Sclera: _____

Cornea: _____

Palpation

Lacrimal glands: _____

Eyelids: _____

Eyeballs: _____

Ophthalmoscope Exam

	Right Eye	**Left Eye**
Red reflex		
Retina		
Optic disc		
Macula		
Vessels		
Lesions		

Comments: _____

_____

_____

NCLEX®-STYLE REVIEW QUESTIONS

Read each question carefully. Choose the best answer for each question.

1. In which environment is mydriasis most likely to occur?
   1. A movie theater
   2. A park
   3. An examination room
   4. A swimming pool

2. The nurse knows that which of the following is(are) true about the conjunctiva? (Select all that apply.)
   1. Lines the interior of the eyelids
   2. Produces a lubricating fluid
   3. Protects the eye
   4. Is normally red in color
   5. Is not responsive to pain

3. The nurse is aware that there are _____ extraocular muscles for each eye.
   1. four
   2. five
   3. six
   4. eight

4. Which of the following questions would be necessary when conducting a focused interview related to the eye? (Select all that apply.)
   1. "Have you ever been diagnosed with diabetes?"
   2. "Have you ever been diagnosed with hypertension?"
   3. "Have you ever been diagnosed with multiple myeloma?"
   4. "Have you ever been diagnosed with glaucoma?"
   5. "Have you ever been diagnosed with urticaria?"

5. A 1-year-old appears to have "cross eyes." The nurse explains this problem to the mother by stating it can be caused by:
   1. trauma at birth
   2. antiseizure medication she was taking during pregnancy
   3. an eye infection when the baby was born
   4. weakness of the eye muscle

6. During the ophthalmoscope exam on a client with hyperopic vision, the nurse should rotate the diopter wheel to:
   1. minus numbers
   2. plus numbers
   3. There are no numbers on the diopter wheel
   4. Plus and minus numbers are irrelevant to hyperopic vision

7. When using the ophthalmoscope to inspect a client's ocular fundus, the nurse understands that it is best to:
   1. begin with the diopter on –10
   2. rotate the wheel to the plus numbers if the client's vision is myopic
   3. approach the client from a 15-degree angle toward the client's nose
   4. rotate the wheel to the minus numbers if the client's vision is hyperopic

8. The nurse is aware that the condition in which the refraction of light is spread over a wide area rather than on a distinct point on the retina is called:
   1. strabismus
   2. astigmatism
   3. retinal detachment
   4. glaucoma

9. A first grader is brought to the school nurse because he was hit in the eye with a ball during recess. After assessing the client, the nurse documents periorbital edema of the right eye. Periorbital edema refers to:
   1. swelling of the soft tissue surrounding the eye
   2. inversion of the lid and lashes
   3. redness around the cornea
   4. a papular appearance of the lower lid

10. The nurse is aware that the leading cause of blindness in the United States is:
    1. glaucoma
    2. congenital birth defects
    3. diabetic retinopathy
    4. chronic eye infections

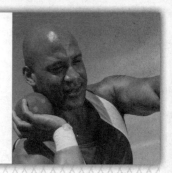

16 Ears, Nose, Mouth, and Throat

Knowing is not enough; we must apply. Willing is not enough; we must do.
—Bruce Lee

The ears, nose, mouth, and throat are important structures of the head and neck. Assessment of these structures provides valuable information about the health of the respiratory and neurologic systems and the abdomen with which they are related. This chapter focuses on methods and techniques to gather and analyze subjective and objective data related to the ears, nose, mouth, and throat.

OBJECTIVES

At the completion of these exercises, you will be able to:

1. Review the anatomy and physiology of the ears, nose, mouth, and throat.
2. Select the equipment necessary to complete an assessment of the ears, nose, mouth, and throat.
3. Identify the correct techniques for assessment of the ears, nose, mouth, and throat.
4. Analyze subjective and objective data related to the assessment of the ears, nose, mouth, and throat.
5. Recognize factors that can influence assessment findings.

6. Apply critical thinking in analysis of a case study.
7. Assess the ears, nose, mouth, and throat on a laboratory partner.
8. Document an assessment of the ears, nose, mouth, and throat.
9. Complete NCLEX®-style review questions related to assessment of the ears, nose, mouth, and throat.

ANATOMY & PHYSIOLOGY REVIEW

1. For each of the following diagrams, label the structures as indicated by each line.

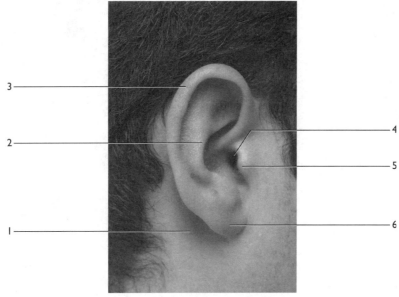

External ear

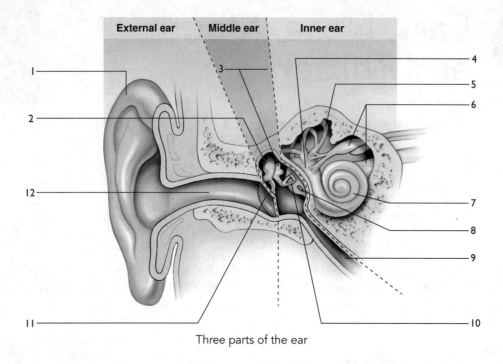

Three parts of the ear

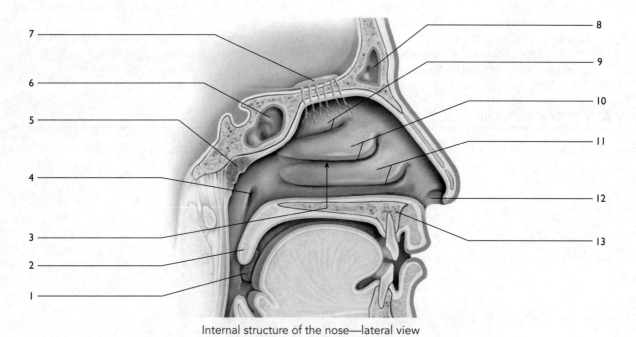

Internal structure of the nose—lateral view

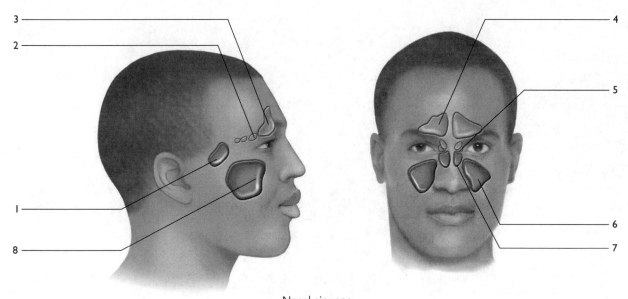

Nasal sinuses

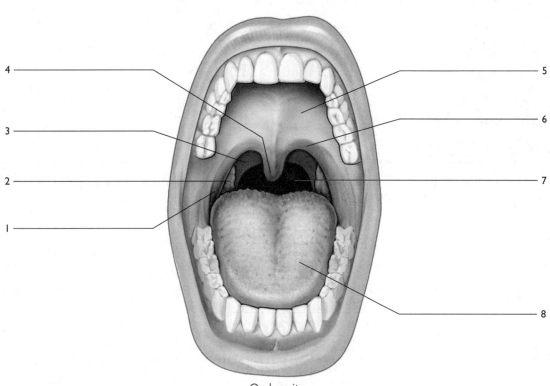

Oral cavity

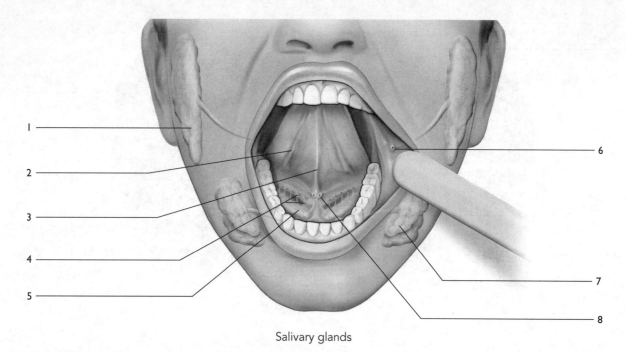

Salivary glands

2. Using the numbers 1 through 10, identify the pathway of sound waves through the structures below, as sound travels from the external ear to the brain. Next, circle all of the structures that are included in the middle ear.

_____ Malleus	_____ Cranial nerve VIII
_____ Cochlea	_____ Auditory canal
_____ Auditory cortex	_____ Incus
_____ Pinna	_____ Oval window
_____ Stapes	_____ Tympanic membrane

EQUIPMENT SELECTION

Prior to beginning the physical assessment of a client's ears, nose, mouth, and throat, it is important to gather the appropriate assessment equipment. Place a check mark next to each piece of equipment that you would need to perform this assessment.

EQUIPMENT		
Cotton balls	Lubricant	Sphygmomanometer
Cotton-tipped applicator	Nasal speculum	Stethoscope
Culture media	Ophthalmoscope	Tape measure
Dental mirror	Otoscope	Test tubes
Doppler ultrasonic stethoscope	Penlight	Thermometer
Examination gown	Reflex hammer	Tongue blade
Eye cover	Ruler	Transilluminator
Flashlight	Skinfold calipers	Tuning fork
Gauze	Skin-marking pen	Vaginal speculum
Gloves	Slides	Vision chart
Goggles	Specimen containers	Watch with second hand
Goniometer	Speculum covers	Wood's lamp

ASSESSMENT TECHNIQUES

Review each assessment technique. If the technique is correct, circle the number. If the technique is incorrect, write the correct assessment technique on the line provided.

1. After palpating the auricle, the nurse should push on the tragus.

_____

_____

2. To perform an otoscopic examination, the nurse should use the largest speculum that fits most comfortably in the auditory canal.

_____

_____

3. When inspecting the auditory canal of an adult client with the otoscope, the nurse should pull the pinna up, back, and out.

_____

_____

4. The nurse uses only one monosyllable word when performing the whisper test.

_____

_____

5. The nurse is assessing a client's hearing and places the tuning fork on the angle of the mandible in order to assess bone conduction during the Rinne test.

_____

_____

6. The nurse places the tuning fork at the midline of the posterior portion of the frontal bone during the Weber test.

_____

_____

7. During the Romberg test, the nurse asks the client to stand with feet together and eyes closed.

_____

_____

8. When using a nasal speculum, the nurse should stabilize the client's head with his or her dominant hand.

_____

_____

9. The nurse palpates the maxillary sinuses by pressing his or her thumbs below the client's superior orbital ridge.

_____

_____

10. When inspecting a client's salivary glands, the nurse should look for the Stensen's ducts near the frenulum.

_____

_____

11. To assess a client's throat, the nurse asks the client to say "aah" and then uses the tongue blade to depress the middle of the arched tongue enough to clearly visualize the throat.

_____

_____

ASSESSMENT FINDINGS

Read each assessment finding. Identify the finding as normal or abnormal by writing an "N" for normal or an "A" for abnormal on each line provided.

_____ 1. Bone conduction longer than tympanic air conduction during the Rinne test

_____ 2. Moist cerumen

_____ 3. Negative Romberg test

_____ 4. Dark pink nasal mucosa

_____ 5. Erythema to tympanic membrane

_____ 6. Smooth vascular ventral surface of tongue

_____ 7. Symmetrical lips

_____ 8. Sweet, fruity breath

_____ 9. Midline nasal septum

_____ 10. Patent external auditory meatus of ear

_____ 11. White patches on membrane

_____ 12. Lateralized sound during the Weber test

_____ 13. Equal-sized nares

_____ 14. Maxillary sinus tenderness

_____ 15. Movable tragus

_____ 16. Absence of red glow from transillumination of the sinuses

_____ 17. Hard palate intact

_____ 18. Exudate in posterior pharynx

_____ 19. Patent nares

_____ 20. Gingival hyperplasia

FACTORS THAT INFLUENCE PHYSICAL ASSESSMENT FINDINGS

Fill in the blank to complete each statement.

1. The auditory canal in infants has a/an _____ curve.

2. Hyperemia of the sinuses in the pregnant female may lead to _____ and _____.

3. Gradual hearing loss in the older adult is called _____.

4. Salivation begins at _____ months of age.

5. The hair at the opening of the auditory meatus becomes more _____ with age.

6. Cerumen in the Asian and Native American cultures may appear _____ in consistency and _____ in color.

7. Clients who participate in activities that increase exposure to loud sounds or music are at increased risk for _____.

8. Cleft lip and palate occur with greatest frequency in the _____ culture.

9. Tics, jaw clenching, and lip biting are all common behaviors that may be assessed in a client who has been experiencing _____.

10. Tooth decay is _____ common among Caucasians.

APPLICATION OF THE CRITICAL THINKING PROCESS

Read the scenario below and then answer the questions that follow in the space provided.

Kenny is a 2-year-old boy who stuck cotton-tipped swabs in both his ears and ran around the house. Unfortunately, he tripped over the dog and hit his head on the stairs. His mother rushed to him as he began to scream. She became extremely alarmed when she pulled the cotton-tipped swab out of his left ear and noted blood. She immediately took him to his healthcare provider's office.

1. List five focused interview questions the nurse should ask.

   1.

   2.

3.

4.

5.

2. With the potential of a perforated tympanic membrane, should the nurse perform the otoscope examination? Explain.

3. Is it necessary to assess Kenny's hearing? Explain.

ASSESSMENT AND DOCUMENTATION

Perform an ears, nose, mouth, and throat assessment on your lab partner and document your findings on the following documentation form.

EARS, NOSE, MOUTH, AND THROAT

Name:_____Date:_____

Age: _____ Gender: _____

FOCUSED INTERVIEW

Reason for today's visit _____

_____

EARS

General Questions

Describe your hearing. Have you noticed any change in your hearing? _____

If so, have the changes been gradual or sudden? _____

Have you noticed a hearing loss of certain sounds or tones, or all hearing? _____

_____

Do you notice hearing loss when using a telephone? Watching television? During conversations? _____

_____

When was your last hearing test? _____

Does you hearing seem better in one ear than the other? If so, which ear is better? _____

_____

Has any member of your family had ear problems or hearing loss? _____

Have you ever been diagnosed with a disease affecting the ears? _____

If so, when were you diagnosed? What treatment was prescribed for the problem? What kinds of things do you do to help with the problem? Has the problem ever recurred? How are you managing the disease now?

_____

Do you now have or have you had an ear infection? _____

If so, when were you diagnosed? What treatment was prescribed? Was the treatment helpful? What kinds of things do you do to help with the problem? Has the problem ever recurred? How are you managing the

infection now? _____

Have you had any ear drainage? If so, describe it. _____

Have you had dizziness, nausea, vomiting, or ringing in your ears? _____

_____

Do you have any pain in your ears? _____

How do you clean your ears? _____

Do you either own or use a hearing aid? _____

Are you taking any medications? What are they? How often do you take them? _____

_____

Are you frequently exposed to loud noises? When? How often? Are protective devices available and do

you use them? _____

_____

Do you experience ear infections or irritations after swimming or being exposed to dust or smoke? If so,

describe them. _____

_____

Age-Related Questions

Infants and Children

Does the child have recurrent ear infections? How many ear infections has the child had in the last 6 months? How were they treated? Has the child had any ear surgery such as insertion of ear tubes?

When? What were the results? Does the child attend day care? _____

_____

_____

Does the child tug at his/her ears? Does the child respond to loud noises? If the child is over 6 months of age, does the child babble? Have you ever had the child's hearing tested? What were the results? Has the child had measles, mumps, or any disease with a higher fever? Has the child been treated recently with any

antibiotics such as streptomycin or neomycin? How do you clean the child's ears? _____

_____

_____

Pregnant Females

Have you ever experienced a ringing in your ears? Have you experienced an earache or a feeling of fullness in your ears? _____

_____

Older Adults

Do you wear a hearing aid? If so, is it effective? How often do you wear your hearing aid? Do you have any difficulty operating the hearing aid? How do you clean the hearing aid? _____

_____

NOSE AND SINUSES

General Questions

Are you having any problems with your nose or sinuses? If so, describe them. Are you able to breathe through your nose? Can you breathe through both nostrils? Is one side obstructed? Describe any problems you have had breathing in the past few days or in the past few weeks. _____

_____

_____

Do you have nasal discharge? If so, is it continuous or occasional? Describe the discharge. _____

_____

Do you have nosebleeds? How often? What is your usual blood pressure? Do you use nasal sprays? How do you treat your nosebleeds? _____

_____

Have you ever had any nose injury or nose surgery? If so, describe it. How was the injury treated? Do you have any residual problems from the injury or surgery? _____

_____

Describe your sense of smell. Are there any circumstances, objects, places, or activities that affect your sense of smell? If so, describe them. _____

_____

What prescription or over-the-counter drugs do you take to relieve your nasal symptoms? Do you use a nasal inhalant, oxygen, or a humidifier to help you breathe? What other medications do you take regularly?

_____

_____

Do you use recreational drugs? If so, what drugs? How often? _____

_____

Age-Related Questions

Infants and Children

Does the child put objects into his/her nose? Does the child frequently have drainage from the nose?

_____

_____

Pregnant Females

Have you had nosebleeds during your pregnancy? If so, how often? _____

_____

MOUTH AND THROAT

General Questions

How would you describe the condition of your mouth and teeth? Have you noticed any changes in the past few months? _____

_____

Do you have any problems swallowing? _____

Do you have any sores or lesions in your mouth or on your tongue? If so, describe them. Are they present constantly or do they come and go periodically? _____

_____

Do your gums bleed frequently? _____

Have you noticed a change in your sense of taste recently? _____

What dental problems, surgeries, or procedures have you had in the past? Please describe in detail.

_____

_____

Do you wear dentures, partial plates, retainers, or any other removable or permanent dental appliance? Does it fit well? Is it comfortable? Why are you wearing the appliance? Does it help resolve the problem?

Are any of your teeth capped? Which ones? _____

_____

How often do you brush your teeth or dentures? Do you use floss regularly? _____

_____

When was your last dental examination? Are you unable to eat some foods because of problems with your teeth? Do you have any pain in one or more teeth? _____

_____

Do you have frequent sore throats? _____

Have you noticed any hoarseness or loss of your voice? _____

Do you now or did you ever smoke a pipe, cigarettes, or cigars? Chew tobacco or dip snuff? How much? How often? _____

Age-Related Questions

Infants and Children

Does the child suck his/her thumb or a pacifier? _____

When did the child's teeth begin to erupt? _____

Does the child go to bed with a bottle at night? What is in the bottle? _____

Does the child know how to brush his/her teeth? Does the child brush daily? _____

How often does the child go to the dentist? _____

Is the child's drinking water fluoridated? _____

Older Adults

Are you able to chew all types of food? _____

Do you experience dryness in your mouth? _____

Do you wear dentures? If so, do they fit properly? _____

PHYSICAL ASSESSMENT

Vital signs: _____ BP _____ HR _____ RR _____ Temp

EAR

Does the client hear the questions asked? Did the client answer appropriately? _____

_____

Inspection

Symmetry:	Right: _____	Left: _____
Proportion:	Right: _____	Left: _____
Color:	Right: _____	Left: _____
Integrity:	Right: _____	Left: _____
Discharge, redness, swelling, lesions, or nodules	Right: _____	Left: _____

Palpate

Auricle and tragus for swelling, nodules, pain, or lesions	Right: _____	Left: _____
Mastoid process for swelling, nodules, pain, or lesions	Right: _____	Left: _____

Inspect

Auditory canal for tenderness, inflammation, lesions, growths, discharge, or foreign substances	Right: _____	Left: _____
Amount, color, and texture of cerumen	Right: _____	Left: _____
Tympanic membrane color, presence of cone-shaped reflection	Right: _____	Left: _____
Whisper test	Right: _____	Left: _____
Rinne test	Right: AC: ____ BC: ____	Left: AC: ____ BC: ____

Weber test _____

Romberg test _____

NOSE AND SINUSES

Inspection of Nose

Symmetry: Frontal: _____   Lateral: _____

Size: Frontal: _____   Lateral: _____

Shape: Frontal: _____   Lateral: _____

Skin lesions: Frontal: _____   Lateral: _____

Signs of infection: Frontal: _____   Lateral: _____

Confirm the nose is straight, in proportion to the other facial structures, midline, and without deformities; the nares are equal in size; the skin is intact; and no drainage or inflammation is present.

Patency   Right: _____   Left: _____

Palpate

External nose for tenderness,
swelling, and stability   Right: _____   Left: _____

Inspect

Vestibule and inferior turbinates
for color, swelling, discharge,
bleeding, polyps, or foreign
bodies   Right: _____   Left: _____

Palpate

Frontal and maxillary sinuses
for discomfort or pain   Right: _____   Left: _____

Percuss

Frontal and maxillary sinuses
for discomfort or pain   Right: _____   Left: _____

Transilluminate the sinuses—
frontal and maxillary   Right: _____   Left: _____

MOUTH AND THROAT

Inspect

Inspect and palpate the lips for
symmetry, color, lesions, texture,
and moisture   Right: _____   Left: _____

Inspect teeth, noting overall dental hygiene; note any occlusion when client clinches teeth _____

_____

Note any dentures and caps; any loose, broken, misaligned, or missing teeth; inflamed gums; and color

of teeth _____

_____

Inspect and palpate the buccal mucosa, gums, and tongue _____

_____

Have client touch the roof of the mouth with the tip of the tongue to note the ventral surface; palpate the tongue and under the tongue for lesions or nodules _____

_____

Inspect the mucous lining of the mouth and gums; note the integrity of the soft and hard palate; inspect the frenula of the tongue, the upper lip, and the lower lip _____

_____

Inspect the salivary glands, Wharton's ducts, and Stensen's ducts; note any pain, tenderness, swelling, or redness _____

Confirm the flow of saliva from the salivary ducts _____

Inspect the throat, uvula, soft palate, and tonsils; note color of the structures and any mouth odors

_____

NCLEX®-STYLE REVIEW QUESTIONS

Read each question carefully. Choose the best answer for each question.

1. The nurse knows that the eustachian tube connects the middle ear with what structure?
   1. Cochlea
   2. Vestibule
   3. Nasopharynx
   4. Sphenoid sinus

2. The nurse encourages parents to begin dental checkups for children beginning at what age?
   1. As soon as the first tooth erupts
   2. 3–4 years
   3. 6–7 years
   4. Once the child loses the first deciduous tooth

3. The nurse knows that taste buds are innervated by what nerves?
   1. Trigeminal and facial nerves
   2. Facial and glossopharyngeal nerves
   3. Olfactory and vagus nerves
   4. Glossopharyngeal and hypoglossal nerves

4. A certified nurse midwife is caring for a client who is 28 weeks pregnant and complaining of sinus pressure and a runny nose. The nurse recognizes that these common complaints during pregnancy are due to what situation?
   1. Elevated estrogen levels causing hyperemia to the sinuses
   2. Elevated progesterone levels causing hyperemia to the sinuses
   3. A decreased immune response
   4. These are not common complaints during pregnancy

5. An older adult presents to a community health center with "ringing in her ears." Which of the following questions would be appropriate for the nurse to ask during the focused interview? (Select all that apply.)
   1. "What medications have you been taking?"
   2. "Are you exposed to loud noises?"
   3. "Have you felt dizzy or nauseated?"
   4. "Do you have any pets at home?"
   5. "Do you have dentures?"

6. An adult client presents to the community health center complaining of nasal congestion, sore throat, and fever. The nurse takes the client's history and performs a physical assessment. Which of the following findings should the nurse record in the subjective section of the client's chart? (Select all that apply.)
    1. Oral temperature 101.5°F
    2. Difficulty swallowing
    3. Pharynx with erythema
    4. Throat pain 5 (scale 0–10)
    5. Nighttime chills

7. If the nurse is unable to visualize the tympanic membrane during the otoscope examination, what should the nurse do next?
    1. Reposition the auricle with the otoscope in place
    2. Remove the otoscope, reposition the auricle, and reinsert the otoscope
    3. Move on to the other ear and document "unable to identify" in the notes
    4. Seek urgent care for the client because the tympanic membrane is most likely ruptured

8. An adolescent is having his hearing checked by the school nurse. What would the following findings represent to the nurse?
    Weber test—no lateralization
    Rinne test—AC 15 sec, BC 15 sec Right ear
    AC 30 sec, BC 15 sec Left ear
    1. Sensorineural hearing loss in the right ear
    2. Conductive hearing loss in the left ear
    3. Conductive hearing loss in the right ear
    4. All findings are within the expected range

9. The nurse is assessing a client suffering from seasonal allergies. What would the nurse expect the nasal mucosa to look like?
    1. Swollen and red
    2. Swollen and pink
    3. Bleeding
    4. Pale and boggy

10. A mother frantically carries her toddler into the emergency department, stating he fell down a flight of stairs and hit his head multiple times. The child is lethargic and pale. Upon a thorough assessment, it is noted that the tympanic membrane has a bluish tinge to it. How would the nurse note this finding?
    1. A perforated tympanic membrane
    2. Epistaxis
    3. Hemotympanum
    4. A normal finding

17 Respiratory System

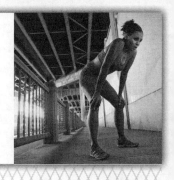

Keep breathing.
—Sophie Tucker

The exchange of oxygen and carbon dioxide is essential for proper functioning of all body systems. The ability of the nurse to recognize subtle changes related to the respiratory status of the client through physical assessment can prevent acute, chronic, and life-threatening situations. This chapter will focus on gathering both subjective and objective data related to the respiratory assessment, as well as analysis of the data collected.

OBJECTIVES

At the completion of these exercises, you will be able to:

1. Review the anatomy and physiology of the respiratory system.
2. Identify the correct techniques for assessment of the respiratory system.
3. Analyze subjective and objective data related to assessment of the respiratory system.
4. Recognize factors that can influence assessment findings.
5. Apply critical thinking in analysis of a case study.
6. Relate objectives in *Healthy People 2020* to the assessment of the respiratory system.
7. Assess the respiratory system on a laboratory partner.
8. Document an assessment of the respiratory system.
9. Complete NCLEX®-style review questions related to the assessment of the respiratory system.

ANATOMY & PHYSIOLOGY REVIEW

1. For each of the following diagrams, label the structures as indicated by each line.

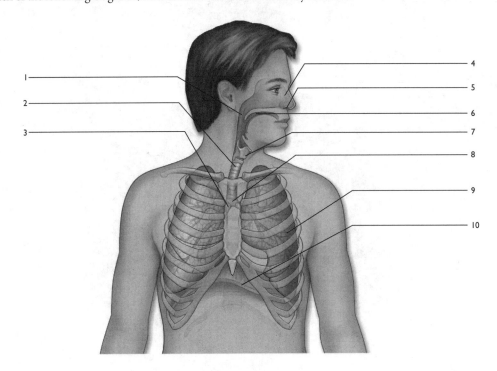

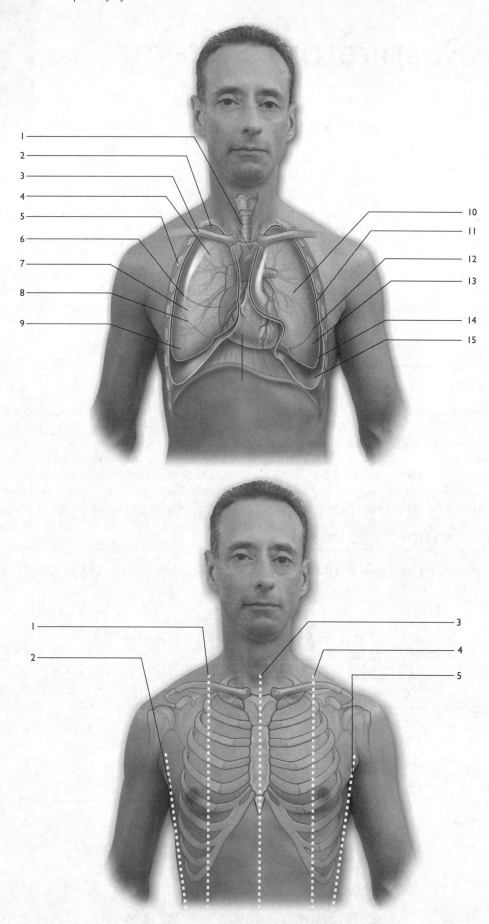

1
2
3
4
5
6
7
8
9

10
11
12
13
14
15

1
2

3
4
5

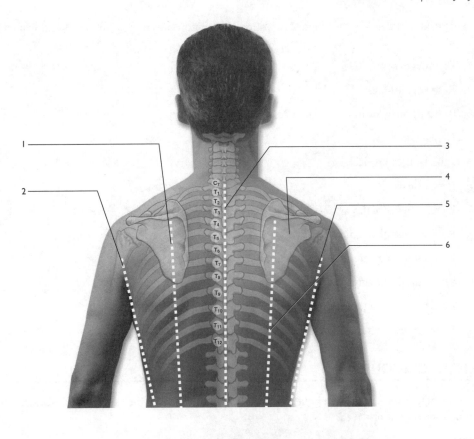

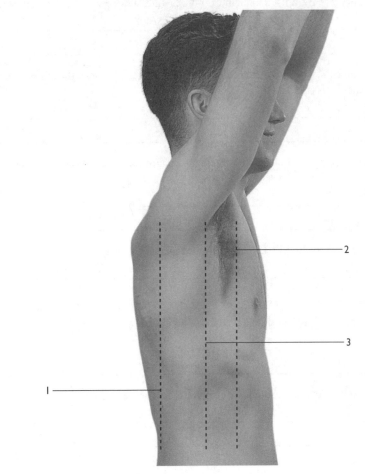

2. Read each statement. Write an "I" if the action occurs during inspiration and an "E" if it occurs during expiration on the line provided.

_____ 1. Diaphragm contracts

_____ 2. Recoil of the lungs

_____ 3. Contraction of the intercostal muscles

_____ 4. Diaphragm relaxes

_____ 5. Alveolar pressure decreases

_____ 6. Lung expansion

_____ 7. Increase in size of thoracic cavity

_____ 8. Passive phase of breathing

_____ 9. Relaxation of the intercostal muscles

_____ 10. Rise of the diaphragm

_____ 11. Decrease in size of thoracic cavity

_____ 12. Diaphragm lowers

ASSESSMENT TECHNIQUES

Review each assessment technique. If the technique is correct, circle the number. If the technique is incorrect, write the correct assessment technique on the line provided.

1. When counting a respiratory rate, the nurse should inform the client that he or she is counting the rate.

   _____

   _____

2. When palpating and counting the ribs and intercostal spaces of the posterior thorax, the nurse should instruct the client to flex the neck, round the shoulders, and lean forward.

   _____

   _____

3. The nurse can palpate for respiratory expansion by placing the palmar surface of his or her hands on the posterior lower chest of the client.

   _____

   _____

4. The ulnar surface of the hand or the finger pads can be pressed against the chest wall to assess tactile fremitus.

   _____

   _____

5. During percussion of the thorax, the client should hold his or her breath.

   _____

   _____

6. During percussion of the thorax, the nurse should begin at the apices of the lungs.

   _____

   _____

7. To properly assess for diaphragmatic excursion, the nurse should begin to percuss at the level of T7 or T8 of the vertebral column.

_____

_____

8. When auscultating lung sounds, the nurse should move the stethoscope to the next area after listening through a full respiratory cycle.

_____

_____

9. When auscultating voice sounds using egophony, the nurse should ask the client to say "ninety-nine" each time the stethoscope is placed on the thorax.

_____

_____

10. Assessment of the anterior thorax is not performed with female clients who have a large amount of breast tissue because of interference in sound perception.

_____

_____

ASSESSMENT FINDINGS

Read each assessment finding. Identify the finding as normal or abnormal by writing an "N" for normal or an "A" for abnormal on each line provided.

_____ 1. Pallor of skin
_____ 2. Symmetrical chest movement
_____ 3. Firm muscle mass over thorax
_____ 4. Vibrations over chest wall while client speaks
_____ 5. Respiratory rate of 26 in an adult
_____ 6. Unilateral delay in chest expansion
_____ 7. Eupnea
_____ 8. Costal angle less than 90 degrees
_____ 9. Atelectasis
_____ 10. Anterior/posterior diameter equal to the transverse diameter

_____ 11. Midline sternum
_____ 12. Even height of scapulae
_____ 13. Posterior thorax nontender
_____ 14. Vesicular sounds between the scapulae
_____ 15. Pink undertones of skin for Caucasians
_____ 16. Resonance on percussion of lung fields
_____ 17. Intercostal muscle retraction
_____ 18. Stridor
_____ 19. Bibasilar rales
_____ 20. Lateral deviation of thoracic spinous process

FACTORS THAT INFLUENCE PHYSICAL ASSESSMENT FINDINGS

Fill in the blank to complete each statement.

1. During fetal development gas exchange occurs at the _____.
2. The respiratory rate _____ from infancy into childhood.
3. During the third trimester of pregnancy, it is common for eupnea to change to _____.
4. There is less expansion of the _____ cavity in the older adult.
5. Oxygen consumption can increase by _____% throughout pregnancy.
6. The heating and cooling ducts in office buildings may carry airborne organisms that cause workers to have frequent respiratory _____.

7. Children in _____ socioeconomic groups have a higher incidence of asthma.

8. In the infancy period, the lateral and anterior-posterior diameters of the chest are _____.

9. Costal breathing is expected after _____ years of age.

10. The costal angle _____ during pregnancy.

11. As altitude increases, the partial pressure of oxygen _____.

12. Forced hot air heating systems can cause _____ to membranes of the body.

Respiratory Patterns

Match the name of each wave pattern in Column A with its associated waveform in Column B by writing the waveform's letter on the line provided.

Column A

_____ 1. Cheyne-Stokes

_____ 2. Hyperventilation

_____ 3. Bradypnea

_____ 4. Eupnea

_____ 5. Tachypnea

_____ 6. Eupnea with a sigh

_____ 7. Hypoventilation

_____ 8. Obstructive breathing with prolonged expiration

Column B (Waveforms)

A.

B.

C.

D.

E.

F.

G.

H.

Auscultation Review

1. Using the diagram below, place an X over each area where the nurse should place the stethoscope when auscultating breath sounds. Then number the Xs in the order in which you will proceed. Provide a rationale for your pattern.

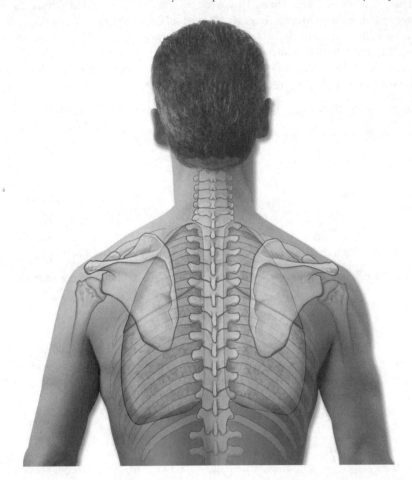

Auscultation Pattern Rationale: _____

_____

2. Match the auscultated sound in Column A with the description in Column B by writing the description's letter on the line provided.

Column A

_____ 1. Crackles

_____ 2. Stridor

_____ 3. Vesicular

_____ 4. Egophony

_____ 5. Bronchophony

_____ 6. Bronchial

_____ 7. Wheeze

_____ 8. Friction rub

_____ 9. Rhonchi

_____ 10. Bronchovesicular

_____ 11. Tracheal

_____ 12. Whispered pectoriloquy

Column B

A. Inspiration louder than expiration
B. Moist bubbling sound
C. "EEEEEEEE" or "AAAAAA"
D. Grating, rubbing sound
E. Continuous snoring/rattling sound
F. Inspiration equal to expiration
G. Harsh, high-pitched sound
H. "Ninety-nine"
I. High-pitched, shrill sound
J. "One, two, three"
K. Loud crowing sound
L. Expiration greater than inspiration

APPLICATION OF THE CRITICAL THINKING PROCESS

Read the scenario below and then answer the questions that follow in the space provided.

Keith is a 20-year-old male who plays guitar in a band. He is 6 feet tall and weighs 165 lb. His medical-surgical history indicates an appendectomy at age 14 and an allergy to citrus fruits. He has been smoking one to two packs of cigarettes per day for about 3 years and admits to occasionally smoking marijuana (about two to three times per month). During a concert performance with his band, he suddenly felt a pain under his left rib cage. He began to experience shortness of breath and thought for a second he was going to faint. He quickly ran off the stage and sat down in a back room. A friend ran to his side and noticed that Keith was having some difficulty breathing and called for medical assistance.

When presenting in the emergency department, Keith's vital signs were BP 142/90, HR 120, RR 36, and T 99.2°F (tympanic).

1. List three focused interview questions the nurse should ask Keith at this time:

   1.

   2.

   3.

During a pain assessment, the nurse collects the following data: The client experienced a sudden onset of pain under his left rib cage that he rated as an 8 on the numeric pain scale; taking a deep breath makes the pain worse.

2. Using the OLDCART & ICE acronym, list any information that has not been collected regarding the pain assessment.

3. Upon physical assessment, it is noted that Keith's skin color is pale and his breathing is rapid and labored. His chest expansion is asymmetrical, and he has absent breath sounds in his left lower lobe. His oxygen saturation level is 91% on room air. Upon collecting this data, the nurse must determine if Keith should be seen by the doctor immediately or if he can wait in the waiting area. State what the nurse's decision should be and provide a rationale.

4. After careful assessment and diagnostic testing, it is determined that Keith has a spontaneous pneumothorax of his left lung.
   1. Define pneumothorax.

   2. List three assessment findings from the above data that support this medical diagnosis.

      1.

      2.

      3.

5. Write nursing diagnoses for Keith in this scenario using NANDA or the PES method.
   1. Nursing diagnosis: _____

   2. Nursing diagnosis: _____

6. Using your presented nursing diagnoses, write an anticipated outcome. How would you evaluate this outcome?

HEALTHY PEOPLE 2020

Read the Healthy People 2020 *objective and answer the questions that follow in the space provided.*

A *Healthy People 2020* objective is:

Reduce the number of workdays missed among persons with current asthma.

1. List four asthma triggers.

   1.

   2.

   3.

   4.

2. Discuss how an occupational health nurse can use this objective to promote and maintain health and function of the respiratory system among employees.

ASSESSMENT AND DOCUMENTATION

Perform an assessment of the respiratory system on your lab partner and document your findings on the following documentation form.

RESPIRATORY SYSTEM

Name:_____Date:_____

Age: _____ Gender: _____

FOCUSED INTERVIEW

Reason for today's visit: _____

_____

General Questions

Describe your breathing today: _____

Do you breathe through your mouth or nose? _____

Describe any changes in your breathing in the past:

   2 days: _____

   2 weeks: _____

   2 months: _____

   2 years: _____

Allergies: _____

     Respiratory symptoms: _____

Recent illness: _____

Current medical conditions: _____

Medication: _____

     Prescription: _____

     OTC: _____

Tobacco use, marijuana use, or any herbal products: _____

Flu immunization: _____

Pneumonia immunization: _____

Describe any disorders you have related to your lung function: _____

_____

_____

Describe any disorders your family members have related to lung function: _____

_____

_____

Symptoms or Behaviors

Do you now or have you ever had:

     Cough: _____

     Mucus/phlegm: _____

     Hemoptysis: _____

     Shortness of breath: _____

     Orthopnea: _____

     Pain/discomfort: _____

          O

          L

          D

          C

          A

          R

          T

          I

          C

          E

Age-Related Questions

Infants and Children

Eating solid foods? Y/N Describe: _____

# of colds in past 12 months: _____

Immunization: _____

Describe safety measures taken at home: _____

Pregnant Females

Shortness of breath? Y/N Describe:_____

Dyspnea? Y/N Describe: _____

Older Adults

Describe any changes in breathing: _____

Difficulty performing daily activities: _____

More tired than usual? Describe: _____

Immunizations: _____

Environment

Allergies: _____

Respiratory irritant exposure: _____

Recent travel out of the country? _____

PHYSICAL ASSESSMENT

Vital signs: _____ BP _____ HR _____ RR _____ Temp

Inspection of the Thorax

Skin color: _____

Nail bed color: _____

Thorax shape: _____

Symmetry: _____

Movement: _____

Use of accessory muscles: _____

Nasal flaring: _____

Breathing pattern: _____

Posture: _____

Palpation of the Thorax

Muscle mass: _____

Lumps/nodules: _____

Tenderness: _____

Respiratory expansion: _____

Tactile fremitus: _____

Percussion

Anterior thorax: _____

Posterior thorax: _____

Diaphragmatic excursion: _____

Auscultation

Anterior thorax

Breath sounds: _____

Vesicular: _____

Bronchovesicular: _____

Bronchial: _____

Tracheal: _____

Adventitious: location and describe

Posterior thorax

Breath sounds: _____

Vesicular: _____

Bronchovesicular: _____

Bronchial: _____

Tracheal: _____

Adventitious: location and describe

Voice Sounds

Bronchophony: _____

Egophony: _____

Whispered pectoriloquy: _____

COMMENTS: _____

_____

_____

NCLEX®-STYLE REVIEW QUESTIONS

Read each question carefully. Choose the best answer for each question.

1. The nurse identifies the structures of the lower respiratory tract as:
   1. the pharynx, bronchi, and lungs
   2. the trachea, bronchi, and lungs
   3. the sinuses, larynx, and bronchi
   4. the larynx, bronchi, and lungs

2. The nurse understands the action associated with expiration is:
   1. a contraction of respiratory muscles
   2. chest expansion
   3. a decrease in alveolar pressure
   4. a decrease in negative intrapleural pressure

3. The nurse identifies signs of respiratory distress to include: (Select all that apply.)
   1. circumoral cyanosis
   2. respiratory rate of 22
   3. intercostal muscle retractions
   4. nasal flaring
   5. periorbital edema

4. A 19-year-old female arrives at the university clinic complaining of asthma-like symptoms. The nurse would most likely hear which of the following sounds upon auscultation?
   1. Loud, moist, bubbling sounds
   2. Low-pitched, grating sounds
   3. High-pitched, continuous sounds
   4. Crackling sounds

5. When auscultating for bronchophony, the nurse should instruct the client to:
   1. repeat the letter "E"
   2. repeat the number "ninety-nine"
   3. repeat the words "one, two, three"
   4. take a deep breath and hold it

6. An adult male client has suffered from emphysema for approximately 5 years. When percussing his posterior lung fields, the nurse is most likely to hear:
   1. hyperresonance
   2. dullness
   3. flatness
   4. resonance

7. Which client would most likely have the largest measured diaphragmatic excursion?
   1. A 22-year-old runner
   2. A 68-year-old smoker
   3. A 3-year-old
   4. A 35-year-old female who is 32 weeks pregnant

8. When auscultating lung sounds, which of the following assessment findings would require further investigation by the nurse? Inspiration is:
   1. greater than expiration over the peripheral lung fields
   2. less than expiration over the trachea
   3. equal to expiration at the sternal border between the scapulae
   4. greater than expiration over the trachea

9. During a focused interview, the nurse asks the client if she sleeps using two or three pillows. This question is important because the client may: (Select all that apply.)
1. snore
2. experience orthopnea
3. be prone to respiratory infections if she is sleep deprived
4. be obese
5. have a history of deep venous thrombosis

10. The nurse identifies the following muscles as accessory muscles for respiratory function. (Select all that apply.)
1. Trapezius
2. Scalene
3. Sternocleidomastoid
4. Pectorals
5. Gracilis

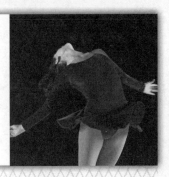

18 > Breasts and Axillae

Patience and perseverance have a magical effect before which difficulties disappear and obstacles vanish.

—John Quincy Adams

Breasts are unique to the individual. They go through many changes throughout each month based on hormone fluctuations, weight fluctuations, and some medications. The ability of the nurse to recognize these changes through assessment and educate clients to perform their own assessments is crucial in early diagnosis of disease. This chapter will focus on gathering both subjective and objective data related to the breast and axillae assessment, as well as analysis of the data collected.

OBJECTIVES

At the completion of these exercises, you will be able to:

1. Review the anatomy and physiology of the breasts and axillae.
2. Identify the correct techniques for assessment of the breasts and axillae.
3. Analyze subjective and objective data related to assessment of the breasts and axillae.
4. Recognize factors that can influence assessment findings.
5. Apply critical thinking in analysis of a case study.
6. Relate objectives in *Healthy People 2020* to the breasts and axillae.
7. Assess the breasts and axillae on a laboratory partner.
8. Document an assessment of the breasts and axillae.
9. Complete NCLEX®-style review questions related to the assessment of the breasts and axillae.

ANATOMY & PHYSIOLOGY REVIEW

1. For each of the following diagrams, label the structures as indicated by each line.

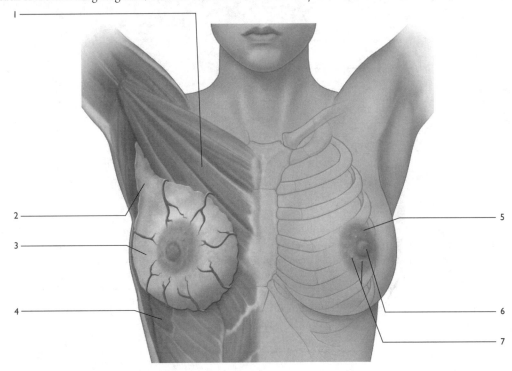

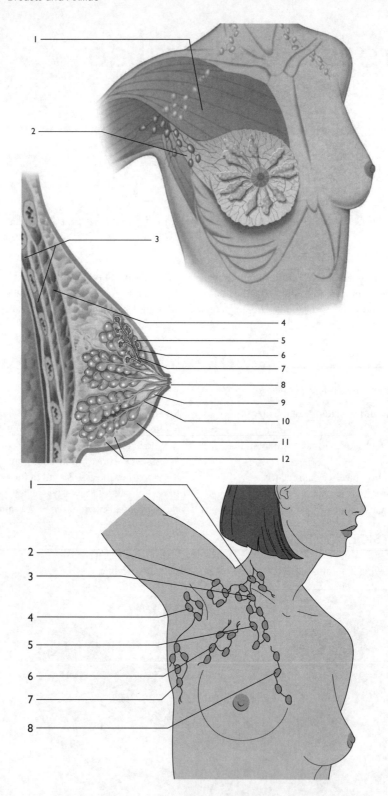

2. Place a check mark [✔] next to each statement that is **TRUE** about the physiology of the breast. If the statement is **FALSE** rewrite the statement correctly in the space provided.

_____   1. Breast tissue starts to change at the onset of puberty between the ages of 14 and 16.

Correction: _____

_____   2. Decreased levels of progesterone and increased levels of estrogen cause changes in fat deposits, ductile maturity, and pigmentation of the breasts.

Correction: _____

_____ 3. Breast growth may be asymmetrical.

Correction: _____

_____ 4. Each breast has 5 to 10 lobes of glandular tissue.

Correction: _____

_____ 5. Acini cells produce milk that is emptied into the lactiferous ducts and carried to the nipple.

Correction: _____

_____ 6. Each breast lobe is composed of 20 to 40 lobules.

Correction: _____

_____ 7. Blood is supplied to the breasts by the Montgomery artery.

Correction: _____

_____ 8. Spence glands are sebaceous glands that produce oils to lubricate and moisturize the areola and nipple.

Correction: _____

ASSESSMENT TECHNIQUES

Review each assessment technique. If the technique is correct, circle the number. If the technique is incorrect, write the correct assessment technique on the line provided.

1. The client should be in a supine position at the beginning of a breast assessment.

_____

_____

2. Explain to the female client that at least three positions will be used during the assessment of the breasts.

_____

_____

3. Inspection of the breasts can be done with the client's hands pressed together at the level of the waist.

_____

_____

4. Inspection of the breasts can be done with the client leaning back on the exam table.

_____

_____

5. When palpating one breast, the nurse should cover the breast that is not being examined.

_____

_____

6. The nurse should place a small pillow or rolled towel under the breast that is not being examined.

_____

_____

7. The finger pads of the first three fingers should be used in a slightly rotary motion during palpation of the breast.

_____

_____

8. The only pattern that covers the entire breast is the concentric circle pattern.

_____

_____

9. If a female client has pendulous breasts, the nurse should place one hand under the breast to support it while the other hand is palpating.

_____

_____

10. The nipple should be compressed between the second and third digit.

_____

_____

ASSESSMENT FINDINGS

Read each assessment finding. Identify the finding as normal or abnormal by writing an "N" for normal or an "A" for abnormal on each line provided.

_____ 1. Dimpling

_____ 2. Oval areolae

_____ 3. Nipple discharge

_____ 4. Presence of axillary hair

_____ 5. Nonpalpable axillary lymph nodes

_____ 6. Unilateral areola tenderness

_____ 7. Inverted nipples for 2 weeks

_____ 8. Pendulous breasts

_____ 9. Bilateral venous patterns

_____ 10. Breasts fall freely and evenly when sitting or standing

_____ 11. Peau d'orange

_____ 12. Slight asymmetry of breasts

_____ 13. Smooth skin over the breast

_____ 14. Galactorrhea

_____ 15. Gynecomastia

_____ 16. Uninterrupted breast contour

_____ 17. Firm pectoral muscles

_____ 18. Thick breast skin

_____ 19. Red, scaly areolae

_____ 20. Supernumerary nipple

FACTORS THAT INFLUENCE PHYSICAL ASSESSMENT FINDINGS

Fill in the blank(s) to complete each statement.

1. Swollen breast tissue in a newborn may be caused by _____.

2. In the female, fatty tissue will replace _____ tissue at menopause.

3. Research has suggested that a high-fat diet may _____ a female's risk of developing breast cancer.

4. Infants may produce a thin discharge from the breasts known as _____ _____. This secretion will subside as the maternal _____ decreases.

5. Women with very small, very large, or asymmetrical breasts are at higher risk for _____ disturbance.

6. The nipples become _____ and _____ in the older adult.

7. Asian and Hispanic women have the _____ rates of breast cancer.

8. During pregnancy, the nipples and areolae become _____ in color and _____ in size.

9. Many women avoid doing _____ because their culture has prohibited looking at or touching oneself.

10. Adolescent male "breast buds" usually disappear within _____ of onset.

THE BREAST SELF-EXAM (BSE)

Fill in the blanks to complete each sentence. Next, number the steps of the breast self-exam in the order in which a nurse would teach a female client to perform them, with 1 being the first step and 10 being the last.

_____ Compare breasts for _____, _____, _____, and _____.

_____ Observe the breasts in front of a/an _____.

_____ Many women palpate their breasts while they _____.

_____ Examine the nipples for _____ and recent _____.

_____ Palpation of the breast should be done with the _____ _____.

_____ Observe the breasts in _____ positions.

_____ Instruct the client to palpate from the periphery of the breasts to the _____.

_____ Compress the nipple with the _____ and _____.

_____ A technique for palpation of the breasts is _____ _____.

_____ Instruct the client not to forget the _____ _____.

APPLICATION OF THE CRITICAL THINKING PROCESS

Read the scenario below and then answer the questions that follow in the space provided.

Jill is a 34-year-old female gravida 3 para 2. She delivered a healthy baby 5 weeks ago and is breastfeeding with support from a lactation nurse at the hospital. Last night, Jill began feeling extremely fatigued, but attributed this to lack of sleep, as her newborn is up several times at night to breastfeed. She also noticed a slight burning sensation when the baby fed from her left breast last night, and today she notes that the breast is slightly swollen and tender. She is concerned that something might be wrong and calls the lactation nurse at the hospital.

1. What three focused interview questions could the lactation nurse ask this client?

   1. _____
   2. _____
   3. _____

The lactation nurse asks Jill to come to the hospital for an assessment. Inspection reveals the breasts are asymmetrical, with the left being larger than the right and with slightly reddened skin. The left breast is warm, firm, and tender to the touch. The areola appears cracked and tender. The nurse assesses Jill's vital signs, which reveal BP 104/68, HR 102, RR 18, and Temp 100.8°F (orally).

2. Identify three assessment findings found during inspection.

   1. _____
   2. _____
   3. _____

3. Identify three assessment findings found during palpation.

   1. _____
   2. _____
   3. _____

The nurse begins to assess Jill's pain by asking about the exact location of the pain, when the pain began, and for the client to rate the pain on a numeric scale. Jill states the discomfort started the previous evening and rated her pain as a 6 on a numerical scale of 0 to 10.

4. Document the pain-related data collected using the OLDCART & ICE pain assessment.

5. What questions should be asked to complete the pain assessment?

The lactation nurse suspects that Jill has developed mastitis of the left breast from a clogged milk duct. The nurse places a call to the healthcare provider for prescriptive treatment. Jill expresses concern that she could have prevented this from happening. The lactation nurse determines that Jill could benefit from education about measures to prevent mastitis.

6. Write one teaching goal and three objectives for this scenario.

   Goal:

   Objectives:

   1.

   2.

   3.

HEALTHY PEOPLE 2020

Read the Healthy People 2020 *objective and answer the questions that follow in the space provided.*

A Healthy People 2020 *objective is:*

> **Increase the proportion of women ages 40 years and older who have received
> a breast cancer screening based on the most recent guidelines.**

1. What is included in a breast cancer screening?

2. Discuss how a women's health nurse can use this *Healthy People 2020* objective to promote and maintain health and function of the client's breasts.

ASSESSMENT AND DOCUMENTATION

Perform a breast and axillae assessment on your lab partner and document your findings on the following documentation form.

BREASTS AND AXILLAE

Name:_____Date:_____

Age: _____ Gender: _____

FOCUSED INTERVIEW

Reason for today's visit: _____

_____

General Questions

Describe the condition of your breasts today: _____

Describe any changes in your breasts in the past:

     2 weeks: _____

     2 months: _____

     2 years: _____

Last menstrual period: _____

     How many days is your menstrual cycle? _____

     Describe any changes in your menstrual cycle: _____

     Describe any breast changes during your menstrual cycle: _____

Allergies: _____

Recent illness: _____

Current medical conditions: _____

Medications: _____

Past surgeries related to the breasts: _____

Describe any disorders you have related to your breasts: _____

_____

Describe any breast disorders your family members have had: _____

_____

When was your last mammogram? _____

     Findings: _____

     Do you perform breast self-exams? _____

     How often? _____

     Findings: _____

Have you had a breast exam performed by a healthcare provider? _____

     How often? _____

     Findings: _____

Describe your current exercise routine: _____

     What type of bra do you wear when you exercise? _____

Do you use any deodorant/antiperspirant/powder under or around your breasts and axillae? _____

_____

Describe how you feel about your breasts. _____

_____

Symptoms or Behaviors

Do you now or have you ever had:

     Lumps: _____

     Discharge: _____

Rashes: _____

Skin changes: _____

Pain/discomfort: _____

       O
       L
       D
       C
       A
       R
       T
       I
       C
       E

Age-Related Changes

Preadolescents

Describe any changes in size or shape of breasts: _____

Describe how you feel about your breasts and the way they are changing: _____

Pregnant Females

Describe changes noticed since last exam: _____

Older Adults

Describe changes noticed in your breasts: _____

PHYSICAL ASSESSMENT

Breast

Inspection

Sitting

Size:	Right: _____	Left: _____
Shape:	Right: _____	Left: _____
Symmetry:	Right: _____	Left: _____
Color:	Right: _____	Left: _____
Venous pattern:	Right: _____	Left: _____
Moles/markings:	Right: _____	Left: _____
Areolae		
Color:	Right: _____	Left: _____
Texture:	Right: _____	Left: _____
Characteristics:	Right: _____	Left: _____

Nipples

    Color: Right: _____   Left: _____

    Texture: Right: _____   Left: _____

    Characteristics: Right: _____   Left: _____

Arms Over Head

Size: Right: _____   Left: _____

Shape: Right: _____   Left: _____

Symmetry: Right: _____   Left: _____

Surface: Right: _____   Left: _____

Suspensory ligaments: Right: _____   Left: _____

Hands Pressed Against Waist

Size: Right: _____   Left: _____

Shape: Right: _____   Left: _____

Symmetry: Right: _____   Left: _____

Surface: Right: _____   Left: _____

Suspensory ligaments: Right: _____   Left: _____

Hands Pressed Together at Waist Level

Size: Right: _____   Left: _____

Shape: Right: _____   Left: _____

Symmetry: Right: _____   Left: _____

Surface: Right: _____   Left: _____

Suspensory ligaments: Right: _____   Left: _____

Leaning Forward from Waist

Size: Right: _____   Left: _____

Shape: Right: _____   Left: _____

Symmetry: Right: _____   Left: _____

Surface: Right: _____   Left: _____

Suspensory ligaments: Right: _____   Left: _____

AXILLAE

Skin: Right: _____   Left: _____

Color: Right: _____   Left: _____

Texture: Right: _____   Left: _____

Hair distribution: Right: _____   Left: _____

Lumps: Right: _____   Left: _____

Lesions: Right: _____   Left: _____

Palpation

Breasts

Tissue characteristics: Right: _____   Left: _____

Lumps: Right: _____   Left: _____

Thickness: Right: _____   Left: _____

Tenderness: Right: _____   Left: _____

Firmness: Right: _____   Left: _____

Nipple

    Texture: Right: _____   Left: _____

    Discharge: Right: _____   Left: _____

Areolae

    Texture: Right: _____   Left: _____

Node enlargement: Right: _____   Left: _____

AXILLAE

Texture: Right: _____   Left: _____

Lumps: Right: _____   Left: _____

Lesions: Right: _____   Left: _____

Tenderness: Right: _____   Left: _____

Nodes: Right: _____   Left: _____

Comments: _____

_____

_____

NCLEX®-STYLE REVIEW QUESTIONS

Read each question carefully. Choose the best answer for each question.

1. The nurse notes speckled raised areas on the areolas of a female client. What is the nurse's best action?
    1. Notify the healthcare provider
    2. Attempt to squeeze the serous glands
    3. Apply topical steroid cream
    4. Document as sebaceous glands

2. A male newborn has milky white discharge from the nipples. What is the nurse's best action?
    1. Notify the healthcare provider
    2. Assure the parents this will resolve in a couple weeks
    3. Retake the child's temperature
    4. Auscultate the lungs for signs of respiratory infection

3. A school nurse is teaching a group of young girls about puberty. The nurse explains that breast tissue will begin to enlarge during puberty between the ages of:
    1. 7 and 10
    2. 9 and 13
    3. 12 and 16
    4. 14 and 18

4. A male client refuses a breast exam by the nurse. What is the nurse's first action?
   1. Inform the client that breast cancer can occur in males as well as females
   2. Document the client's refusal
   3. Continue with the remainder of the assessment
   4. Refer the client for a mammogram

5. Which statement by the nurse best explains changes in breast tissue during menopause? The breast tissue experiences:
   1. an increase in glandular tissue
   2. a decrease in fatty tissue
   3. relaxation of the suspensory ligaments
   4. an increase in erectile sensitivity to the nipple

6. A 14-year-old girl is having an annual physical. She appears quite embarrassed during the examination and shyly asks the nurse if it is normal for one of her breasts to be larger than the other. The nurse's response should be:
   1. "Breast development may not be the same on both sides; this is quite normal"
   2. "We will schedule you for a breast ultrasound"
   3. "Let's find out if your mother's breasts are the same way"
   4. "Do you have a history of breast cancer in the family?"

7. A nurse is working in a health and wellness center on a university campus. She was asked by a sorority to give a presentation during Breast Cancer Awareness month. In the presentation, the nurse decides to include which of the following guidelines from the American Cancer Society?
   1. Women in their 20s have an option to perform a monthly breast self-exam (BSE)
   2. A breast exam should be performed by a healthcare provider every 5 years after the age 25
   3. All females should have a baseline mammography at age 50
   4. All females over age 40 should perform a BSE once per week

8. A 19-year-old female college student just finished reading an article in a fashion magazine on breast cancer. It really upset her, because her aunt died of breast cancer 2 years ago. The student decides that it is time for her to start thinking about performing breast self-examination (BSE). Unsure of what to do, she consults the nurse at the college health service. The nurse includes which of the following statements regarding BSE?
   1. "It is best to perform BSE about 5 days prior to your menstrual period"
   2. "It is best to perform BSE about 5 days after your menstrual period"
   3. "It is best to perform BSE during your menstrual period"
   4. "You don't have to worry about BSE at your age."

9. The nurse knows that the incidence of breast cancer in the female is highest in the:
   1. axillary tail
   2. upper inner quadrant
   3. lower outer quadrant
   4. lower inner quadrant

10. Which of the following would the nurse document as an abnormal assessment finding during the menstrual cycle?
   1. Breast tenderness
   2. Breast pain
   3. Breast swelling
   4. Nipple discharge

19 Cardiovascular System

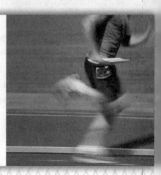

There is no instinct like that of the heart.
—Lord Byron

The cardiovascular system is responsible for the continuous circulation of blood throughout the body. The physiology of the cardiac cycle consists of blood flow and electrical conduction. Understanding this cycle is an important aspect in performing a complete cardiovascular assessment. This chapter will focus on gathering both subjective and objective data related to the cardiovascular system, as well as analysis of the data collected.

OBJECTIVES

At the completion of these exercises, you will be able to:

1. Review the anatomy and physiology of the cardiovascular system.
2. Identify the correct techniques for assessment of the cardiovascular system.
3. Analyze subjective and objective data related to assessment of the cardiovascular system.
4. Recognize factors that can influence assessment findings.
5. Apply critical thinking in analysis of a case study.
6. Relate objectives in *Healthy People 2020* to the cardiovascular system.
7. Assess the cardiovascular system on a laboratory partner.
8. Document an assessment of the cardiovascular system.
9. Complete NCLEX®-style review questions related to the assessment of the cardiovascular system.

ANATOMY & PHYSIOLOGY REVIEW

1. For each of the following diagrams, label the structures as indicated by each line.

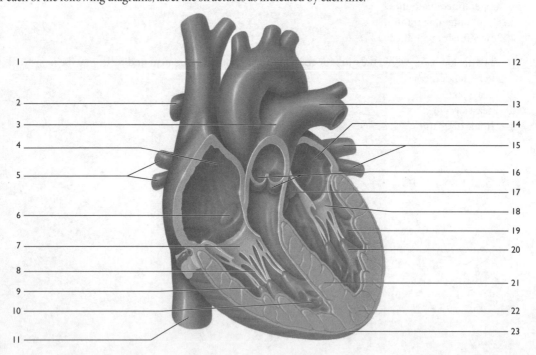

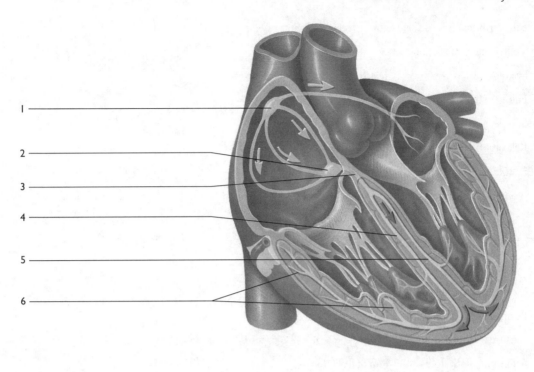

1

2

3

4

5

6

2. Starting with the vena cava, follow a drop of blood through the heart. Place the structures in the boxes provided. Be sure to use proper sequential order.

Aorta	Aortic valve	Left atrium	Left ventricle
Lungs	Mitral valve	Pulmonary artery	Pulmonary vein
Pulmonic valve	Right atrium	Right ventricle	
Tricuspid valve	Vena cava		

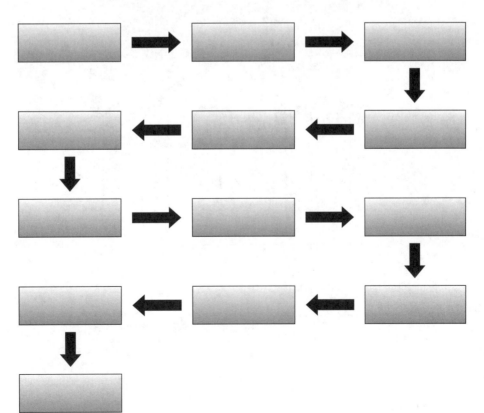

3. Circle the term that is associated with each cardiac event.

    1. Ventricular contraction

       Systole   Diastole

    2. Filling of the ventricles

       Systole   Diastole

    3. Relaxation of the ventricles

       Systole   Diastole

    4. Blood being expelled into the pulmonary artery

       Systole   Diastole

    5. Closure of the tricuspid valve

       Beginning of systole   Beginning of diastole

    6. Closure of the pulmonic valve

       Beginning of systole   Beginning of diastole

    7. Closure of the mitral valve

       Beginning of diastole   End of diastole

    8. Closure of the aortic valve

       Beginning of systole   End of systole

4. Label each part of the ECG.

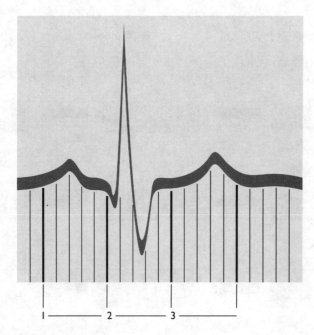

Answer the following questions related to the ECG pattern.

    1. The P wave represents _____.

    2. The P wave lasts _____ seconds.

    3. The QRS interval represents _____.

    4. The QRS interval lasts _____ seconds.

    5. The QT interval represents _____.

6. The QT interval lasts _____ seconds.

7. The PR interval represents _____.

8. The PR interval lasts _____ seconds.

ASSESSMENT TECHNIQUES

Review each assessment technique. If the technique is correct, circle the number. If the technique is incorrect, write the correct assessment technique on the line provided.

1. Begin the assessment of the heart with the client in the supine position.

   _____

   _____

2. Inspection of the cardiovascular system begins with an overview of the general skin color.

   _____

   _____

3. The nail beds should be inspected in the cardiovascular assessment.

   _____

   _____

4. During inspection of the external and internal jugular veins, the nurse should be sure the client's head is turned slightly toward the side being examined.

   _____

   _____

5. When assessing for jugular venous distention, the client should be in a supine position with the head of the examination table elevated to a 45-degree angle.

   _____

   _____

6. When inspecting the chest for pulsations, the client should be in a high-Fowler's position and then a low-Fowler's position.

   _____

   _____

7. Palpate each carotid artery separately.

   _____

   _____

8. When beginning to auscultate heart sounds, the client should breathe normally.

   _____

   _____

9. Initially when auscultating for cardiac murmurs, use the diaphragm of the stethoscope.

   _____

   _____

10. To determine a pulse deficit, the nurse auscultates the apical pulse while simultaneously palpating a carotid pulse.

   _____

   _____

ASSESSMENT FINDINGS

Read each assessment finding. Identify the finding as normal or abnormal by writing an "N" for normal or an "A" for abnormal on each line provided.

_____ 1. Uniform skin color

_____ 2. Bradycardia

_____ 3. Xanthelasma

_____ 4. Apical heart rate of 110 in an adult

_____ 5. Blue nail beds

_____ 6. Precordial heaves

_____ 7. Tetralogy of Fallot in the infant

_____ 8. Patchy hair distribution on legs of adults

_____ 9. QRS interval of 0.08

_____ 10. S1 louder than S2 at the left SB, second ICS

_____ 11. +1 edema in the feet of an adult

_____ 12. Ruddy skin tone

_____ 13. Periorbital edema

_____ 14. Rhythmic head bobbing

_____ 15. Visible carotid pulsations

_____ 16. S3 and S4 in an adult

_____ 17. PR interval of 0.12

_____ 18. Bounding pulse at rest for an adult

_____ 19. Ventricular gallop

_____ 20. S2 louder than S1 at the left MCL, fifth ICS

FACTORS THAT INFLUENCE PHYSICAL ASSESSMENT FINDINGS

Fill in the blank(s) to complete each statement.

1. The _____ _____, a passageway between the atria in the fetus, closes shortly after birth.

2. The blood pressure of a full-term infant is _____ than that of a preterm newborn.

3. Alcoholism may cause ventricular ectopy, which can lead to _____ cardiac output.

4. Cocaine causes a/an _____ in the oxygen demands on the heart.

5. Blood volume may increase as high as _____ % during pregnancy.

6. The most common type of murmur that reveals itself during pregnancy is a/an _____ murmur.

7. Hypertension is most common in the _____ and _____ cultures.

8. Caucasians have _____ serum cholesterol levels than African Americans.

9. The heart walls of an older adult may _____.

10. Ventricular compliance in the older adult may _____.

APPLICATION OF THE CRITICAL THINKING PROCESS

SCENARIO 1

Heena is a 62-year-old Indian female who was brought to the emergency department with dizziness and light-headedness. She states she continues to get a strange sensation in her chest that she cannot describe. Her vital signs are BP 106/52, HR 112, RR 20, and T 98.7 (oral). Heena denies any medical or surgical history. She denies alcohol or tobacco use. She takes an antacid only when she experiences some heartburn, but denies any other medication use.

The nurse immediately places Heena on a cardiac monitor that reveals this rhythm:

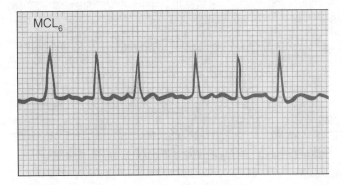

1. Identify the above rhythm: _____

    _____

2. Identify two characteristics of this rhythm.

    1. _____

    2. _____

3. Describe any relationship between the identified rhythm and the client's reports of dizziness and light-headedness.

4. The nurse continues to assess Heena. The nurse asks Heena if she is experiencing any pain at this time; Heena states that she is not. The nurse's next question should be:

5. Heena's heart rate decreases to 89 beats per minute and she indicates she is starting to feel a little better. The cardiologist asks the nurse to monitor the client. List three factors that should be "monitored" during this time.

    1. _____

    2. _____

    3. _____

SCENARIO 2

Earl is an 81-year-old male who was diagnosed with congestive heart failure (CHF) 2 years ago. His condition has been managed by medication and careful monitoring. During his visit to the CHF clinic, the nurse discovers that Earl has gained 4 lb in the past 3 days.

1. Discuss if this is a normal or abnormal finding.

2. List three signs or symptoms that may be associated with congestive heart failure.

    1.

    2.

    3.

Vicki, a student nurse, is spending the day at the CHF clinic. Her preceptor has asked her to check Earl's heart rate. Vicki checks a radial pulse for 30 seconds and multiplies it by 2 and reports her findings to her preceptor. The preceptor appeared to be upset with Vicki's method of collecting this data.

3. What assessment technique would have been appropriate in collecting this data? Provide a rationale.

HEALTHY PEOPLE 2020

Read the Healthy People 2020 *objective and answer the questions that follow in the space provided.*

A *Healthy People 2020* objective is:

Reduce coronary heart disease deaths.

1. Define coronary heart disease.

2. List two risk factors for coronary heart disease that cannot be changed.

   1.

   2.

3. List two risk factors for coronary heart disease that can be changed.

   1.

   2.

4. Discuss how a nurse educator can use this objective to promote and maintain the health and function of the cardiovascular system.

ASSESSMENT AND DOCUMENTATION

Perform a cardiovascular assessment on your lab partner and document your findings on the following documentation form.

CARDIOVASCULAR

Name: _____ Date: _____

Age: _____ Gender: _____

FOCUSED INTERVIEW

Reason for today's visit: _____

_____

General Questions

Describe the condition of your heart today: _____

Describe any changes of your heart in the past:

     2 weeks: _____

     2 months: _____

     2 years: _____

Smoking: _____

     Substance: _____

     Amount: _____

     Duration: _____

     Have you ever tried to stop: _____

Are you exposed to secondhand smoke? _____

What is your current weight? _____

     Describe any changes in your weight in the past year: _____

Describe your salt intake: _____

Describe your everyday diet: _____

Allergies: _____

Current medications (including prescription, over the counter, and herbal supplements): _____

Using any illicit drugs (marijuana, cocaine, etc.): _____

Recent illness: _____

Current medical conditions: _____

Past medical history: _____

Describe any disorders you have related to your heart: _____

_____

Describe any disorders of the heart in your family: _____

_____

When was your last ECG? _____

     Findings: _____

When was your last blood pressure screening? _____

     Findings: _____

When was your last cholesterol screening? _____

     Findings: _____

Describe your level of stress: _____

Describe your exercise: _____

     Patterns: _____

     Routine: _____

     Frequency: _____

     Bra used: _____

Age-Related Questions

Infants and Children

Describe the pregnancy with this child: _____

Did you smoke, take drugs, or drink alcohol during pregnancy? _____

What is the child's energy level? _____

Does the infant take a long time to feed? _____

Does the infant favor squatting rather than sitting up straight? _____

Does the child have symptoms of joint pain, headaches, fever, or respiratory infections? _____

Is the child gaining weight and growing normally? _____

Pregnant Females

History of heart disease? _____

Hypertension during this pregnancy? _____

Swelling of face or hands? _____

Older Adults

Noted any changes in ability to concentrate, remember things, or perform simple mental tasks? _____

Experienced changes in sexual function? _____

Experienced reactions to medications you are taking? _____

Symptoms or Behaviors

Do you now or have you ever had:

    Skin color changes: _____

    Shortness of breath: _____

    Orthopnea: _____

    Coughing: _____

    Dizziness: _____

    Palpitations: _____

    Pain/discomfort: _____

        O

        L

        D

        C

        A

        R

        T

        I

        C

        E

PHYSICAL ASSESSMENT

Vital signs: _____ BP _____ Apical pulse _____ Respiratory rate _____

Inspection

Skin color: _____

Lips: _____

Eyes: _____

    Sclera: Right: _____   Left: _____

    Periorbital area: Right: _____   Left: _____

Head bobbing: _____

Jugular veins: Right: _____   Left: _____

Carotid arteries: Right: _____   Left: _____

Hands and fingers: Right: _____   Left: _____

Chest wall: _____

Palpation

Carotid arteries: _____

Identify the heart sounds at the following areas:

    Aortic: _____

    Pulmonic: _____

    Erb's point: _____

    Tricuspid: _____

    Mitral: _____

    Epigastric area: _____

Percussion

Cardiac border: _____

Auscultation

Carotid arteries: Right: _____   Left: _____

Identify the heart sounds at the following areas:

    Aortic: _____

    Pulmonic: _____

    Erb's point: _____

    Tricuspid: _____

    Mitral: _____

    Epigastric area: _____

Apical pulse:

    Rate: _____

    Rhythm: _____

NCLEX®-STYLE REVIEW QUESTIONS

Read each question carefully. Choose the best answer for each question.

1. Which of the following statements is true about blood flow through the heart?
    1. Blood travels through the pulmonary vein before it travels through the tricuspid valve
    2. Oxygenated blood travels through the pulmonary artery prior to being ejected from the left ventricle
    3. Deoxygenated blood travels through the pulmonic valve into the pulmonary artery
    4. Blood passes through the mitral valve before it passes through the tricuspid valve

2. The cardiac output equation is:
    1. cardiac output = stroke volume × heart rate for 1 minute
    2. cardiac output = stroke volume × body surface area
    3. cardiac output = cardiac index × heart rate for 1 minute
    4. cardiac output = cardiac index × stroke volume

3. A cardiac cycle is completed in:
    1. 0.12 second
    2. 0.2 second
    3. 0.8 second
    4. 1.2 seconds

4. A 34-weeks-pregnant African American female visits the Women's Health Clinic for a routine exam. Her blood pressure reading in the supine position is 162/88. The nurse's next step would be to:
    1. further assess and monitor the client for preeclampsia
    2. further assess and monitor the client for a systolic murmur
    3. provide the client with fluids for obvious dehydration
    4. continue with the routine assessment and obtain her weight

5. A 4-day-old newborn develops cyanosis of the skin and lips. After extensive diagnostic testing, a diagnosis of tetralogy of Fallot is made. The nurse caring for this newborn discovers that the parents have little understanding of what this actually means. The nurse is aware that this condition includes which combination of cardiac defects?
    1. Atrial septal defect, coarctation of the aorta, right ventricular hypertrophy, and pulmonary stenosis
    2. Dextroposition of the aorta, pulmonary stenosis, atrial flutter, and mitral valve prolapse
    3. Atrial septal defect, left ventricular hypertrophy, pulmonary stenosis, and ventricular septal defect
    4. Dextroposition of the aorta, pulmonary stenosis, right ventricular hypertrophy, and ventricular septal defect

6. The nurse would associate which assessment finding with a pulse deficit?
    1. An absent pulse in more than one extremity
    2. An apical pulse of 88 and a carotid pulse of 78
    3. An apical pulse of 88 and a carotid pulse of 88
    4. An apical pulse of 88 and a carotid pulse of 98

7. When assessing for signs of increased central venous pressure, the nurse decides to inspect the jugular veins. With the client lying at a 45-degree angle, the nurse notes that the jugular veins distend 4.1 cm above the sternal angle. The nurse interprets this as:
    1. a normal finding
    2. an abnormal finding but not indicative of increased central venous pressure
    3. an abnormal finding and indicative of increased central venous pressure
    4. inaccurate data due to the fact that the client should have been sitting at a 90-degree angle

8. A middle-age client with high cholesterol asks the nurse about starting an exercise regimen for a healthy heart. The nurse should be sure to mention that:
    1. only aerobic exercise is beneficial to the heart
    2. only nonaerobic exercise is beneficial to the heart
    3. a combination of aerobic and nonaerobic exercise is beneficial to the heart
    4. people who have high cholesterol should not exercise

9. A 36-year-old male is having a comprehensive history and physical performed. Which of the following pieces of data revealed in his medical history are relevant to the cardiac component of this exam?
   1. Splenectomy
   2. Rheumatic fever as a child
   3. Lactose intolerance
   4. Fractured left scapula

10. A nurse on the telemetry unit at a community hospital has been assigned a 45-year-old female with the diagnosis of "atypical chest pain." She is informed in report that the client has mitral valve regurgitation. The nurse understands that upon auscultation of the cardiac sounds of the client, a:
    1. high-pitched, harsh, blowing sound may be revealed
    2. low, rumbling sound may be revealed
    3. soft, blowing sound may be revealed
    4. medium, coarse, clicking sound may be revealed

20 Peripheral Vascular System

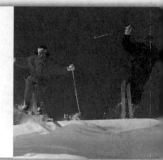

I look to the future because that's where I'm going to spend the rest of my life.
—George Burns

The peripheral vascular system consists of vessels that carry blood throughout the body. High pressures in this system result in hypertension, known as the "silent killer." This chapter will focus on gathering both subjective and objective data related to the peripheral vascular system, as well as analysis of the data collected.

OBJECTIVES

At the completion of these exercises, you will be able to:

1. Review the anatomy and physiology of the peripheral vascular system.
2. Identify the correct techniques for assessment of the peripheral vascular system.
3. Analyze subjective and objective data related to assessment of the peripheral vascular system.
4. Recognize factors that can influence assessment findings.
5. Apply critical thinking in analysis of a case study.
6. Relate *Healthy People 2020* objectives to the peripheral vascular system.
7. Assess the peripheral vascular system on a laboratory partner.
8. Document an assessment of the peripheral vascular system.
9. Complete NCLEX®-style review questions related to assessment of the peripheral vascular system.

ANATOMY & PHYSIOLOGY REVIEW

1. For each of the following diagrams, label the structures as indicated by each line.

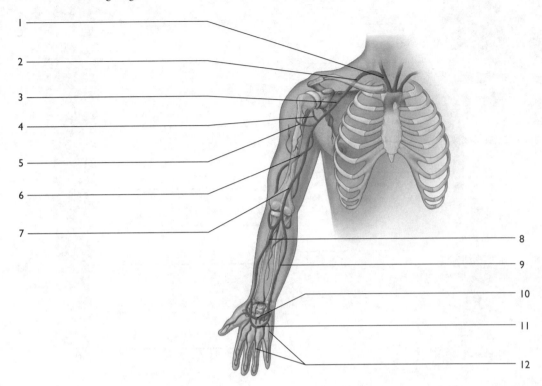

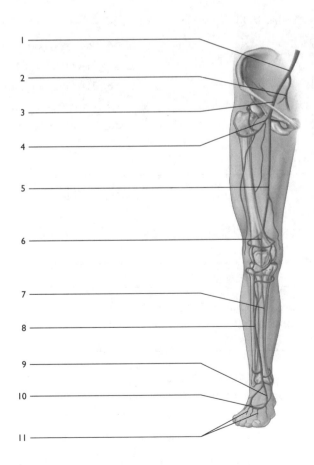

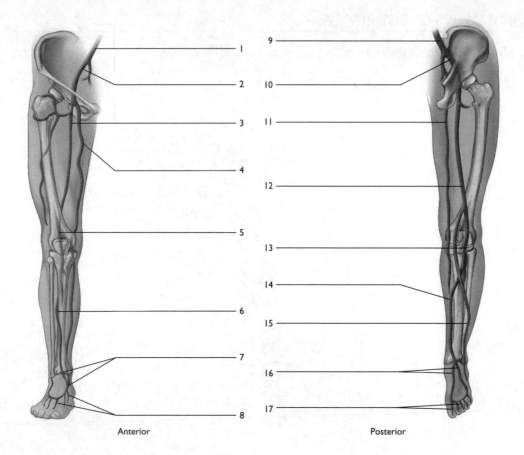

Anterior   Posterior

2. Label each vessel characteristic with a "V" for veins or an "A" for arteries.

_____ **1.** Carry oxygenated blood   _____ **6.** Receive blood from capillaries

_____ **2.** Contain valves   _____ **7.** Have thick walls

_____ **3.** Have thin walls   _____ **8.** Have higher pressure

_____ **4.** Carry blood to the heart   _____ **9.** Carry blood away from the heart

_____ **5.** Carry deoxygenated blood   _____ **10.** Are more elastic

ASSESSMENT TECHNIQUES

Review each assessment technique. If the technique is correct, circle the number. If the technique is incorrect, write the correct assessment technique on the line provided.

1. In the adult, a blood pressure may be obtained on all extremities when performing a complete peripheral vascular assessment.

_____

_____

2. To palpate the carotid artery, the examiner must place the first two or three finger pads between the trachea and the sterno-cleidomastoid muscle and press firmly.

_____

_____

3. To assess for capillary refill, the examiner must apply pressure to one of the client's fingernails for 1 second and then quickly release the pressure.

_____

_____

4. To assess the brachial artery, the examiner must palpate lateral to the biceps tendon.

_____

_____

5. When performing the Allen test, the client should sit with the arms over the head.

_____

_____

6. The epitrochlear lymph node should be easily palpable from behind the elbow to the groove between the biceps and triceps muscles.

_____

_____

7. The manual compression test should be performed with the client standing.

_____

_____

8. During a Trendelenburg test, the tourniquet should be applied around the upper thigh while the client is standing.

_____

_____

9. The client's knee should be flexed 90 degrees while assessing for Homans' sign.

_____

_____

10. If the examiner has difficulty palpating the popliteal artery while the client is supine, the client can rotate to a prone position and flex the knee.

_____

_____

ASSESSMENT FINDINGS

Read each assessment finding. Identify the finding as normal or abnormal by writing an "N" for normal or an "A" for abnormal on each line provided.

_____ 1. Radial pulse 62 bpm in an adult

_____ 2. BP 138/94 in an adult

_____ 3. +2 peripheral pulses in the older adult

_____ 4. Easily palpable epitrochlear node

_____ 5. Warm feet

_____ 6. Positive Homans' sign

_____ 7. Symmetrical popliteal pulses

_____ 8. Yellow, thick toenails

_____ 9. Brachial pulse 102 in an adult

_____ 10. BP 102/62 on an 8-year-old

_____ 11. Regularly irregular rhythm

_____ 12. Capillary refill <2 seconds

_____ 13. Nonpalpable axillary nodes

_____ 14. Necrotic left great toe

_____ 15. Varicosities of the lower extremities

_____ 16. Nonpalpable femoral pulse

_____ 17. +1 dorsalis pedis pulse

_____ 18. Lymphedema

_____ 19. Clubbing of fingernails

_____ 20. Unilateral swelling of the lower extremities

FACTORS THAT INFLUENCE PHYSICAL ASSESSMENT FINDINGS

Fill in the blank(s) to complete each statement.

1. The _____ culture has the highest incidence of hypertension.

2. Individuals of Irish and _____ descent have a greater risk of varicose veins.

3. The arterial walls of an older adult will lose _____.

4. Pressure from the pregnant uterus on the lower extremities obstructs _____ _____.

5. A child over 1 year of age will have a systolic pressure in the thigh that is _____ than that of the arm.

6. Clients with jobs that require standing for most of the day are at greater risk for _____ _____.

7. Hypertension is known as the "silent killer" because it is often _____.

8. Obesity is a risk factor for _____ _____ disease.

9. The _____ of peripheral vascular resistance as a client ages increases the risk of hypertension.

10. In a baby less than 1 year of age, the systolic pressure in the thigh should _____ that of the arm.

Pulse Predicaments

For the conditions listed below, select a pulse or pulses from the list that best describe(s) anticipated findings. Some conditions may have more than one descriptor.

Normal   Pulsus alternans   Pulsus paradoxus   Weak/thready
Absent   Pulsus bigeminus   Unequal pulses   Bounding

1. Aortic regurgitation _____   8. Severe peripheral vascular disease _____

2. Cardiac tamponade _____   9. Cardiac arrest _____

3. Shock _____   10. Systemic hypertension _____

4. Dissecting aneurysm _____   11. Pregnancy _____

5. Pericarditis _____   12. Hyperthyroidism _____

6. Anemia _____   13. Heart failure _____

7. Anxiety _____

Edema

1. Describe the assessment technique that should be used to stage edema.

2. Stage the levels of edema in the diagram below.

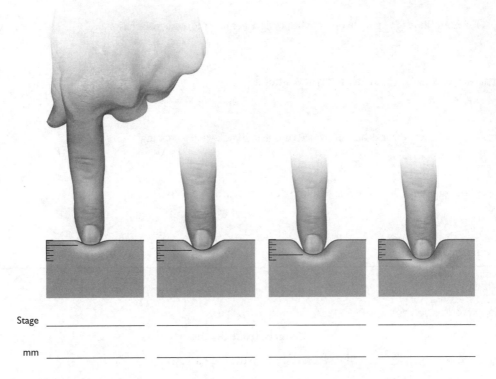

Stage   _____   _____   _____   _____

mm   _____   _____   _____   _____

3. Name three conditions that a client may have if edema is noted.

1.

2.

3.

APPLICATION OF THE CRITICAL THINKING PROCESS

Read the scenario below and then answer the questions that follow in the space provided.

Agnes is a 72-year-old female who was admitted to a medical-surgical unit for a nonhealing wound of her right lateral malleolus. She states it began as a small, circular, discolored lesion that has slowly formed into a pale, nonbleeding, open-centered wound during the past 2 months.

Agnes has a medical history of diabetes, hypertension, and obesity, and she has smoked one pack of cigarettes per day for the past 50 years. Her surgical history is two cesarean sections, a hysterectomy, coronary artery stent placements, and a femoral-popliteal bypass of the left leg 2 years ago that failed and led to a left foot amputation.

Upon admission to the nursing unit, the initial assessment by the nurse notes cool, shiny, pale, hairless skin of both lower legs and thick, brittle, yellow toenails on the right foot. The pedal pulse in the right foot is nonpalpable but faintly audible with the Doppler. The wound is circular, 2 cm in diameter, and has well-defined edges, and the wound bed is a pale yellow with no drainage noted. Agnes states she is in severe pain at 8 on a scale of 1 to 10.

1. Determine if this wound is the result of an arterial or venous problem.

2. Identify signs or symptoms that support your conclusion.

3. What is the best position for Agnes in order to help relieve her pain? Provide your rationale.

4. What risk factors does Agnes have for this type of wound?

5. Is the wound assessment that has been provided complete? If not, what is missing?

6. List at least four questions that the nurse should ask to complete the pain assessment.

HEALTHY PEOPLE 2020

Read the *Healthy People 2020* objective and answer the questions that follow in the space provided.

A *Healthy People 2020* objective is:

Reduce stroke deaths.

1. Stroke is listed as the _____ leading cause of death in the United States.

2. List two risk factors for stroke that cannot be changed (nonmodifiable).

   1.

   2.

3. List two risk factors for stroke that can be changed (modifiable).

   1.

   2.

4. Search the website of a health-related organization to identify the components of two commonly used stroke scales.

   1. Name of scale: _____

   Components of scale

   Site resource (website)

   2. Name of scale: _____

   Components of scale

   Site resource (website)

5. Discuss which stroke scale you prefer. What are the advantages to this scale that helped you make the decision?

6. Discuss how a community health nurse can use this *Healthy People 2020* objective to promote and maintain health and function of the peripheral vascular system.

ASSESSMENT AND DOCUMENTATION

Perform a peripheral vascular assessment on your lab partner and document your findings on the following documentation form.

PERIPHERAL VASCULAR SYSTEM

Name:_____ Date:_____

Age: _____ Gender: _____

FOCUSED INTERVIEW

Reason for today's visit: _____

_____

General Questions

Describe your circulation today: _____

Describe any changes in your circulation in the past:

     2 weeks: _____

     2 months: _____

     2 years: _____

Allergies: _____

Recent illness: _____

Current medical conditions: _____

Past medical history: _____

List current medications (include prescription, over the counter, and herbal supplements):

_____

Describe any disorders you have related to your circulation or lymphatic system: _____

_____

Describe any disorders of the circulation or lymphatic system in your family: _____

_____

Do you smoke? _____

    Substance: _____

    Amount: _____

    Duration: _____

Are you exposed to secondhand smoke? _____

What is your current weight? _____

    Describe any changes in your weight in the past year: _____

When was your last blood pressure screen? _____

    Findings: _____

When was your last cholesterol screening? _____

    Findings: _____

Describe your level of stress: _____

Describe your exercise patterns: _____

    Findings: _____

Describe your current exercise routine: _____

Age-Related Questions

Infants and Children

Has the infant become lethargic? _____

Has the child had a blood pressure screening? _____

Does the child have any enlarged lymph nodes? _____

Pregnant Females

Is your blood pressure being monitored? _____

Any swelling of the face, hands, or legs? _____

Older Adults

No additional questions required.

Symptoms or Behaviors

Skin:

    Color: _____

    Temperature: _____

    Hair distribution: _____

Do you now or have you ever had:

    Swelling: _____

    Sores: _____

Numbness: _____

Tingling: _____

Pain/discomfort: _____

O
L
D
C
A
R
T
I
C
E

PHYSICAL ASSESSMENT

Blood Pressure:

Right arm _____ Left arm _____

CAROTID ARTERIES

Inspection

Pulsations: Right: _____   Left: _____

Palpation

Rate: Right: _____   Left: _____

Rhythm: Right: _____   Left: _____

Amplitude: Right: _____   Left: _____

Apical comparison: _____

Auscultation

Diaphragm: Right: _____   Left: _____

Bell: Right: _____   Left: _____

ARMS

Inspection

Color: Right: _____   Left: _____

Nail beds: Right: _____   Left: _____

Nail bed angle: Right: _____   Left: _____

Palpation

Temperature: Right: _____   Left: _____

Capillary refill: Right: _____   Left: _____

Radial pulse:

    Rate: Right: _____   Left: _____

    Rhythm: Right: _____   Left: _____

    Amplitude: Right: _____   Left: _____

Ulnar pulse:

    Rate: Right: _____   Left: _____

    Rhythm: Right: _____   Left: _____

    Amplitude: Right: _____   Left: _____

Brachial pulse:

    Rate: Right: _____   Left: _____

    Rhythm: Right: _____   Left: _____

    Amplitude: Right: _____   Left: _____

Allen's test: Right: _____   Left: _____

Epitrochlear node: Right: _____   Left: _____

Axillary lymph node: Right: _____   Left: _____

LEGS

Inspection

Color: Right: _____   Left: _____

Hair distribution: Right: _____   Left: _____

Lesions: Right: _____   Left: _____

Edema: Right: _____   Left: _____

Superficial veins: Right: _____   Left: _____

Toenails:

    Color: Right: _____   Left: _____

    Thickness: Right: _____   Left: _____

Palpation

Temperature: Right: _____   Left: _____

Capillary refill: Right: _____   Left: _____

Superficial veins: Right: _____   Left: _____

Manual

compression test: Right: _____   Left: _____

Trendelenburg's test: Right: _____   Left: _____

Homans' sign: Right: _____   Left: _____

Inguinal

Lymph nodes: Right: _____ Left: _____

Femoral pulse:

    Rate: Right: _____ Left: _____

    Rhythm: Right: _____ Left: _____

    Amplitude: Right: _____ Left: _____

Popliteal pulse:

    Rate: Right: _____ Left: _____

    Rhythm: Right: _____ Left: _____

    Amplitude: Right: _____ Left: _____

Dorsalis pedis pulse:

    Rate: Right: _____ Left: _____

    Rhythm: Right: _____ Left: _____

    Amplitude: Right: _____ Left: _____

Posterior tibial pulse:

    Rate: Right: _____ Left: _____

    Rhythm: Right: _____ Left: _____

    Amplitude: Right: _____ Left: _____

Edema: Right: _____ Left: _____

NCLEX®-STYLE REVIEW QUESTIONS

Read each question carefully. Choose the best answer for each question.

1. The nurse identifies which of the following statements as true about veins? Veins:
   1. carry oxygenated blood
   2. have thicker walls than arteries
   3. have one-way intraluminal valves
   4. carry blood away from the heart

2. Which of the following would the nurse consider an average blood pressure for a newborn?
   1. 62/35
   2. 120/80
   3. 100/60
   4. 50 palpable

3. Hypertension is called the "silent killer" because it is often asymptomatic. Which of the following does the nurse identify as symptoms that may be associated with hypertension? (Select all that apply.)
   1. Headache
   2. Epistaxis
   3. Twitching of the eyelids
   4. Chest pain
   5. Palpitations

4. The nurse identifies which of the following clients as **least** likely to develop varicose veins?
   1. 32-year-old hairdresser
   2. 45-year-old trauma nurse
   3. 55-year-old administrative assistant
   4. 26-year-old primigravida

5. Which one of the following questions would be **inappropriate** for the nurse to ask during a focused interview regarding the peripheral vascular system?
    1. "Have you noticed a change in hair growth on your legs?"
    2. "Have you experienced any difficulty in achieving an erection?"
    3. "Do you smoke?"
    4. "Have you noticed any blood in your urine?"

6. The nurse knows that the carotid pulse should be synchronous with:
    1. S1
    2. S2
    3. S3
    4. S4

7. A middle-age client is assisted back to bed after 30 minutes of physical therapy on postoperative day 2 following a left total hip replacement. The client reports pain of 8 out of 10 on the pain scale. The nurse obtains a set of vital signs and notes a radial pulse of 104. The nurse's next step would be to:
    1. notify the doctor because the client is tachycardic
    2. offer the client an analgesic and reassess the vital signs and pain later
    3. notify physical therapy that the sessions should be shorter
    4. allow the client to rest

8. When assessing the carotid pulse of a client in fluid overload, the nurse would expect the amplitude to be:
    1. 0
    2. 1
    3. 2
    4. 3

9. Which of the following tests might the nurse perform if he or she suspects that the client may have a deep venous thrombosis?
    1. Allen's test
    2. Manual compression test
    3. Homans' sign test
    4. Trendelenburg's test

10. An older adult client has a history of venous insufficiency. The client has been admitted to the hospital with an ulcer on the right medial malleolus. The nurse assessing the wound notes which of the following common characteristics of a venous leg ulcer? (Select all that apply.)
    1. Wound is moist and bleeds
    2. Temperature of the skin is cool to the touch
    3. Wound edges are well defined
    4. Deep muscle pain is present
    5. Thickened skin is present around the ankles that may be darker in appearance

21 Abdomen

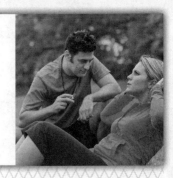

You don't understand anything until you learn it more than one way.
—Marvin Minsky

The abdomen contains organs associated with various body systems. Through a skillful focused interview and physical assessment, the nurse will be able to determine which body systems require further investigation. This chapter will focus on gathering both subjective and objective data related to the assessment of the abdomen, as well as analysis of the data collected.

OBJECTIVES

At the completion of these exercises, you will be able to:

1. Review the anatomy and physiology of the abdomen.
2. Select the equipment necessary to complete the assessment of the abdomen.
3. Identify the correct techniques for assessment of the abdomen.
4. Analyze subjective and objective data related to the assessment of the abdomen.
5. Recognize factors that can influence assessment findings.
6. Apply critical thinking in analysis of a case study.
7. Assess the abdomen on a laboratory partner.
8. Document an assessment of the abdomen.
9. Complete NCLEX®-style review questions related to the assessment of the abdomen.

ANATOMY & PHYSIOLOGY REVIEW

1. For each of the following diagrams, label the structures as indicated by each line.

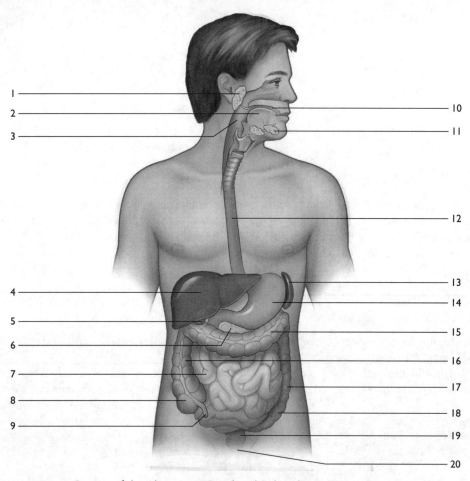

Organs of the Alimentary Canal and Related Accessory Organs

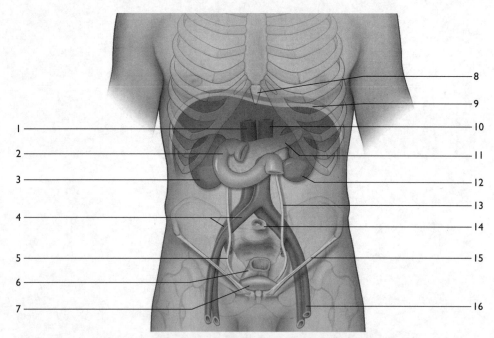

Abdominal Vasculature and Deep Structures

2. Draw lines to map Figure A into four quadrants and Figure B into nine regions. Label each quadrant and region.

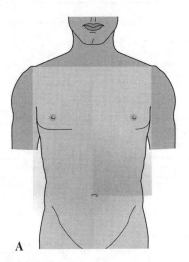

A

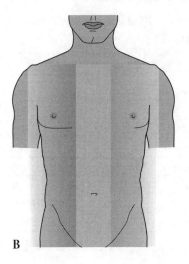

B

3. Place the following structures involved in the digestive process in the correct order from 1 (the first structure involved) through 14 (the last structure involved).

_____ **a.** Anus
_____ **b.** Ascending colon
_____ **c.** Descending colon
_____ **d.** Duodenum
_____ **e.** Esophagus
_____ **f.** Hepatic flexure of the colon
_____ **g.** Ileum

_____ **h.** Jejunum
_____ **i.** Mouth
_____ **j.** Pharynx
_____ **k.** Rectum
_____ **l.** Splenic flexure of the colon
_____ **m.** Stomach
_____ **n.** Transverse colon

4. Identify the location of each of the structures by placing the letter from the provided key on the provided line.

RUQ = Right upper quadrant
RLQ = Right lower quadrant

LUQ = Left upper quadrant
LLQ = Left lower quadrant

_____ **1.** Head of the pancreas
_____ **2.** Sigmoid colon
_____ **3.** Stomach
_____ **4.** Right adrenal gland
_____ **5.** Pyloric sphincter
_____ **6.** Left ovary
_____ **7.** Duodenum

_____ **8.** Left ureter
_____ **9.** Hepatic flexure of colon
_____ **10.** Body of the pancreas
_____ **11.** Appendix
_____ **12.** Spleen
_____ **13.** Gallbladder
_____ **14.** Right spermatic cord

EQUIPMENT SELECTION

Prior to beginning the physical assessment of a client's abdomen, it is important to gather the appropriate equipment. Place a check mark next to each piece of equipment that you would need to perform this assessment.

EQUIPMENT					
	Cotton balls		Lubricant		Sphygmomanometer
	Cotton-tipped applicator		Metric ruler		Stethoscope
	Culture media		Nasal speculum		Tape measure
	Dental mirror		Ophthalmoscope		Test tubes
	Doppler ultrasonic stethoscope		Otoscope		Thermometer
	Drape sheet		Penlight		Tissues
	Examination gown		Reflex hammer		Transilluminator
	Examination light		Skinfold calipers		Tuning fork
	Gauze		Skin-marking pen		Vaginal speculum
	Gloves		Slides		Vision chart
	Goggles		Small pillow		Watch with second hand
	Goniometer		Specimen containers		Wood's lamp

ASSESSMENT TECHNIQUES

Review each assessment technique. If the technique is correct, circle the number. If the technique is incorrect, write the correct assessment technique on the line provided.

1. The client should be in a supine position with a small pillow placed behind the head for assessment of the abdomen.

_____

_____

2. The examination gown should cover the chest and the drape sheet should be placed 1 to 2 inches below the umbilicus.

_____

_____

3. The contour of the abdomen should be assessed at eye level with a light source.

_____

_____

4. The examiner should visualize imaginary horizontal and vertical lines delineating the abdominal quadrants while observing the abdomen.

_____

_____

5. The auscultation pattern for bowel sounds should begin with the right lower quadrant using the diaphragm of the stethoscope.

_____

_____

6. The auscultation pattern for vascular sounds should begin with the femoral arteries.

_____

_____

7. During the abdominal assessment, the examiner should auscultate over the liver and spleen for friction rubs.

_____

_____

8. When percussing the borders of the liver, the examiner should begin at the level of the umbilicus and move toward the rib cage along the extended left midclavicular line.

_____

_____

9. Palpation should occur prior to auscultation in order to avoid changing the natural sounds and movements of the abdomen.

_____

_____

10. Murphy's sign is assessed while the client is lying supine. The examiner can place the right hand above the client's knee. The client is then asked to raise the leg to meet the examiner's hand.

_____

_____

ASSESSMENT FINDINGS

Read each assessment finding. Identify if the finding is normal or abnormal by writing an "N" for normal or an "A" for abnormal on each line provided.

_____ 1. Guarded abdomen

_____ 2. Smooth and moist skin

_____ 3. Hyperactive bowel sounds

_____ 4. Tympany on percussion over the left lower quadrant

_____ 5. Friction rub over RUQ

_____ 6. Renal artery bruit

_____ 7. Rebound tenderness to the LLQ

_____ 8. Hypoactive bowel sounds throughout

_____ 9. Obesity

_____ 10. Venous hum auscultated below the xiphoid process

_____ 11. Rounded abdominal contour

_____ 12. Bulges

_____ 13. Borborygmi

_____ 14. Nonpalpable spleen

_____ 15. Resonance on percussion over the RUQ

_____ 16. Nonpalpable liver

_____ 17. Liver span of 5.5 cm RMCL

_____ 18. Ascites

_____ 19. Pain during the psoas sign

_____ 20. Displaced umbilicus in a 7-months-pregnant female

FACTORS THAT INFLUENCE PHYSICAL ASSESSMENT FINDINGS

Fill in the blank(s) to complete each statement.

1. The umbilical cord consists of _____ artery(ies) and _____ vein(s).

2. Abdominal breathing is seen in the _____ age group.

3. Linea nigra is seen in _____ females.

4. Digestive enzymes _____ in the older adult.

5. Jewish Americans have a greater occurrence of _____ intolerance.

6. The _____ culture is at greater risk for gastric cancer.

7. During pregnancy the _____ enlarges and expands into the abdominal cavity.

8. The older adult and the pregnant female are at risk for _____.

9. Clients who have surgical scars on the abdomen may experience body _____ disturbances.

10. During pregnancy, the fundus of the uterus should be above the pubic bone by week _____.

APPLICATION OF THE CRITICAL THINKING PROCESS

Read each of the scenarios below and then answer the questions that follow in the space provided.

SCENARIO 1

Yvonne is a 36-year-old African American female who delivered a baby boy at 34 weeks' gestation by cesarean section 2 months ago. As Yvonne is changing her baby's diaper, he begins to cry; she notices that he has a lump on his belly. Highly concerned, she calls the pediatrician's office for an appointment.

1. List three focused interview questions the nurse should ask Yvonne upon arrival to the office.

   1.

   2.

   3.

2. The baby's vital signs are BP 75/40, HR 122, RR 38, Temp 99.1°F. Are these stable vital signs for a 2-month-old baby?

3. Upon physical assessment, the nurse notices a ½-inch bulge just below the baby's umbilicus. She reports this finding to the physician. The baby is diagnosed with an umbilical hernia. List two other signs and/or symptoms that may be noted on assessment of the abdomen.

   1.

   2.

4. The baby appears to be comfortable and in no distress. What pain scale would be appropriate for the nurse to use to assess for pain? Provide a rationale.

5. Develop a nursing diagnosis for this baby from the data in the scenario.

SCENARIO 2

Alfonso is a 38-year-old male who arrives at the emergency department complaining of abdominal pain and mild nausea. He has a medical history of irritable bowel syndrome and asthma. He has no surgical history. He has smoked one pack of cigarettes per day for the last 10 years and drinks two to three beers on the weekend.

1. List three focused questions the nurse should ask during this initial interview.

   1.

   2.

   3.

The nurse completes a pain assessment and learns that the pain suddenly started 5 hours ago to the right lower quadrant, is constant, and is a 7 on a 1-to-10 numerical scale. He took three ibuprofen tablets 2 hours ago with no relief.

2. List four questions that should be asked to complete the pain assessment.

   1.

   2.

   3.

   4.

Further data collection reveals the following: BP 142/82, HR 98, RR 20, Temp 101.2°F. Alfonso states he has not had much of an appetite in the past few days. Upon physical assessment, the abdomen is soft and nondistended with positive bowel sounds in all four quadrants. Rebound tenderness is noted in the right lower quadrant, and pain is noted during the psoas test.

3. Alfonso is diagnosed with appendicitis. What assessment factors support this diagnosis?

4. Identify a learning need for this client in the above scenario.

ASSESSMENT AND DOCUMENTATION

Perform an assessment of the abdomen on your lab partner and document your findings on the following documentation form.

ABDOMEN

Name:_____ Date:_____

Age: _____ Gender: _____

FOCUSED INTERVIEW

Reason for today's visit: _____
_____

General Questions

Describe your appetite. Has it changed in the past 24 hours? In the past month? In the past year?
_____
_____

If changed, what do you believe has caused the change in your appetite? Have you done anything to address the change? Have you spoken to a healthcare professional about the change? Has anything else occurred with the change in appetite? _____
_____
_____

Has your weight changed? Over what period of time did the weight change occur? What do you believe has contributed to your weight change? Have any problems or symptoms accompanied the weight change? Have you discussed this with a healthcare professional? _____
_____
_____

Tell me what you have had to eat and drink in the last 24 hours, including snacks. How much of each item did you consume? Is this a typical eating pattern for you? _____
_____
_____

Describe your bowel habits. Describe the color and consistency of your stool._____
_____

Have you experienced any changes in your elimination pattern or in your stool? What kind of change has occurred in your elimination pattern or stool? When did the change begin? Can you identify anything you believe may have caused the change? What have you done about the problem? Have you discussed the changes with a healthcare professional? Are you using laxatives or antidiarrheals at the present time?

Recently in the past? How often? _____
_____
_____

_____

_____

_____

_____

Do you have a feeling of bloating or increased gas? If so, what do you think causes this? Have any changes been made in your diet or medications? What do you do to decrease these feelings? What do you do to relieve the symptoms? Do you use antacids? Do you increase water intake? Do you exercise?

_____

_____

_____

_____

Do you have any physical problems that affect your appetite, affect your bowel functioning, or contribute to abdominal problems? Describe the way your abdominal function is affected. How long has this been occurring? Have you sought relief for the problem? What have you done to relieve the problem? Did the

remedy help? Have you sought advice from a healthcare professional? _____

_____

_____

_____

Is there anyone in your family who has had an abdominal disease or problem? What is the disease or problem? Who in the family now has or has had the disease? When was it diagnosed? Describe the treatment.

How effective was the treatment? _____

_____

_____

_____

Questions Related to Illness or Infection

Have you ever been diagnosed with an abdominal disease? When were you diagnosed with the problem? What treatment was prescribed for the problem? Was the treatment helpful? What kinds of things do you do to help with the problem? Has the problem ever recurred (acute)? How are you managing the disease

now (chronic)? _____

_____

_____

_____

If client is unable to answer specific conditions/diseases in the above question, ask the client about specific conditions/diseases such as cholecystitis, cholelithiasis, ulcers, diverticulosis, and cirrhosis.

_____

_____

Do you now have or have you ever had an infection within the abdomen? When were you diagnosed with the infection? What treatment was prescribed for the problem? Was the treatment helpful? What kinds of things do you do to help with the problem? Has the problem ever recurred (acute)? How are you managing the infection now (chronic)? _____

_____

_____

_____

_____

If client is unable to effectively answer the above question, list possible abdominal disorders such as hepatitis, cholecystitis, and diverticulitis and ask the client to answer yes or no. _____

_____

_____

Questions Related to Symptoms, Pain, and Behaviors

Nausea

Do you have nausea? How long have you had the nausea? How often are you nauseated? Do you know what is causing the nausea? Is there a difference in the nausea at different times of the day? Describe your nausea. Is the nausea accompanied by burning, indigestion, or bloating? _____

_____

_____

_____

_____

Do you vomit when you experience the nausea? What does the vomitus look like? Does the vomitus have any odor? What was the cause, in your opinion? How frequently do you have this experience? What do you do to relieve the symptoms? When you vomit, describe what comes up and the amount.

_____

_____

_____

_____

Do you have pain with the nausea? Have you sought treatment for the nausea? When was the treatment sought? What occurred when you sought that treatment? Was something prescribed or recommended for the nausea? What was the effect of the remedy? Do you use OTC or home remedies for the nausea? What OTC or home remedies do you use? How often do you use them? How much of them do you use?

_____

_____

_____

_____

Do you have any difficulty chewing or swallowing your food? Do you wear dentures? Do you have any crowns? Do your gums bleed easily? Do you have indigestion? _____

_____

_____

Do you suffer from diarrhea or constipation? What do you think is the cause? What have you done to correct the situation? Have these measures helped the situation? Do you experience any rectal itching or bleeding? _____

_____

_____

_____

Pain

Are you having any abdominal pain at this time? Where is the pain? How often do you experience the pain? How long does the pain last? How long have you had the pain? How would you rate the pain on a scale of 0 to 10, with 10 being the worst pain? _____

_____

_____

_____

Does the pain radiate? Where does the pain radiate? Is there a trigger for the pain? Does the pain affect your breathing or any other functions? What do you think is causing the pain? What do you do to relieve the pain? _____

_____

_____

_____

Behaviors

What have you had to eat and drink in the past 24 hours? What snacks do you have in a 24-hour period? What size portions do you eat? Is the 24-hour pattern you described typical for the way you eat? How much coffee, tea, cola, alcoholic beverages, or chocolate do you consume in a 24-hour period?

_____

_____

_____

_____

Age-Related Questions

Infants and Children

Is the baby breastfed or bottle fed? Does the baby tolerate the feeding? How frequently does the baby eat? Have you recently started the baby on any new foods? Is the baby colicky? What do you do to relieve the colic? How much water does the baby drink? _____

_____

_____

_____

Does the toddler eat at regular times? What and how much does the toddler eat? Is the toddler able to feed himself or herself? What type of snacks does the toddler eat? Does the toddler experience restlessness at night related to rectal itching? _____

_____

_____

_____

Is the child toilet trained? Describe how toilet training is taught to the child. Have there been any lapses in toilet training? If so, how frequently? How recently? How do you typically respond to these lapses?

_____

_____

_____

_____

_____

What does the child eat? Does the child bring a lunch and snack to school or buy it at school? When at home, how often does the child snack, and what are the snacks? Does the family have one meal a day together? What kind of food do you eat at this meal? Describe the atmosphere at this meal.

_____

_____

_____

Pregnant Females

Are you experiencing any nausea or vomiting? Are you experiencing any elimination problems such as constipation? Are you experiencing heartburn or flatulence? _____

_____

_____

Older Adults

Are you ever incontinent of feces? How often are you constipated? Do you take laxatives? How often? Which laxative do you take? _____

_____

_____

How many foods containing fiber or roughage do you eat during a typical day? Are you able to get to the store for groceries? Do you eat alone? With someone? _____

_____

_____

Questions Related to the Environment

Internal Environment

How would you describe your stress level? Do you think you are coping well? Could your coping skills be

better? _____

_____

_____

External Environment

Do you work with any chemical irritants? Have you recently done any traveling? Where did you travel?

_____

_____

_____

PHYSICAL ASSESSMENT

Inspection of the Abdomen

As the client is in the supine position with a small pillow placed beneath the head and knees, stand at the right side of the client and observe the client's abdomen. Visualize the quadrants of the abdomen. Determine the contour as flat, rounded, or scaphoid. Observe the position of the umbilicus. Note findings.

_____

_____

Observe skin color of the abdomen and location and characteristics of lesions, scars, and abdominal markings.

Note findings. _____

_____

Observe the abdomen for symmetry, bulging, or masses. Note findings. _____

_____

_____

Observe the abdominal wall for movement. Note findings. _____

_____

Auscultation of the Abdomen

The client remains in the supine position. Tell the client to breathe normally. Using the diaphragm of the stethoscope, auscultate for bowel sounds, starting in the right lower quadrant (RLQ), moving through the other quadrants. Note the character and frequency of the sounds. Count the sounds for at least 60 seconds.

Note findings. _____

_____

_____

Auscultate for vascular sounds using the bell of the stethoscope. Listen at the midline below the xiphoid process for aortic sounds. Move the stethoscope from side to side as you listen over the renal, iliac, and

femoral arteries. Note findings. _____

_____

Auscultate for friction rubs over the abdomen, listening carefully over the liver and spleen. Note findings.

_____

_____

Percussion of the Abdomen

Start percussion in the RLQ of the abdomen and percuss through all of the remaining quadrants. Note findings. _____

_____

Advanced Skill: Percussion of the Liver

Begin percussion at the level of the umbilicus and move toward the rib cage along the extended right midclavicular line (MCL). When the sound along this line changes from tympany to dullness, mark the point with a skin-marking pen. Percuss downward from the fourth intercostal spaced along the right MCL. When the sound changes from resonance to dullness, mark this point with the skin-marking pen. Measure the distance between the two points. This should be approximately 5 to 10 cm. This is known as the liver span. Repeat these steps along the midsternal line, using the same technique. The liver size should to 4 to 9 cm at the midsternal line. To determine the movement of the liver with breathing, ask the client to take a deep breath and hold it. Percuss upward along the extended MCL. The lower liver border should descend about

2.54 cm. Note findings. _____

_____

Advanced Skill: Percussion of the Spleen

Percuss the abdomen on the left side posterior to the midaxillary line; a small area of splenic dullness will usually be heard from the 6th to the 10th intercostal spaces. Note findings. _____

_____

Percussion of the Gastric Bubble

Percuss the abdomen in the area between the left costal margin and the midsternal line extended below the xiphoid process. Note findings. _____

_____

Palpation of the Abdomen

Lightly palpate the abdomen in all four quadrants, starting in the RLQ. Note findings. _____

_____

Deeply palpate the abdomen in all four quadrants, starting in the RLQ. Note findings. _____

_____

Advanced Skill: Palpation of the Liver

While standing on the right side of the client, place your left hand under the lower portion of the ribs. Lift the rib cage with your left hand. Place your right hand into the abdomen using an inward and upward thrust at the costal margin. Note findings. _____

_____

_____

Advanced Skill: Palpation of the Spleen

While standing on the right side of the client, place your left hand under the lower border of the rib cage on the left side and elevate the rib cage. Press the fingers of your right hand into the left costal margin area of the client. While the client is taking slow deep breaths, the diaphragm descends, and the spleen may be palpable if enlarged. Note findings. _____

_____

_____

ADDITIONAL PROCEDURES

Palpate the aorta for pulsations: Using the fingertips, press firmly in the upper abdomen to the left of midline below the xiphoid process. Note findings. _____

_____

TO AVOID CAUSING UNNECESSARY PAIN OR DISCOMFORT, ABDOMINAL PALPATION FOR REBOUND TENDERNESS SHOULD NOT BE PERFORMED WHEN ASSESSING CLIENTS WHOSE CURRENT SUBJECTIVE REPORTS INCLUDE ABDOMINAL PAIN OR TENDERNESS. Palpate for rebound tenderness: Hold hand at a 90-degree angle to the abdominal wall in an area of no pain or discomfort. Press deeply into the abdomen, using a slow and steady movement. Rapidly remove your fingers from the client's abdomen.

Assess the client for pain with this procedure. Note findings. _____

_____

_____

Percuss the abdomen for ascites. Percuss in the midline to elicit tympany. Continue to percuss in lateral directions away from the midline and listen for dullness. Mark the skin, identifying possible levels of fluid.

Measure the abdominal girth with a tape measure. Note findings. _____

_____

_____

Assess for psoas sign when lower abdominal pain is present and appendicitis is suspected. Place your left hand just above the level of the client's right knee. Ask the client to raise the leg to meet your hand. Flexion of the hip causes contraction of the psoas muscle. Note findings. _____

_____

_____

Assess for Murphy's sign by palpating the liver and asking the client to take a deep breath. The diaphragm descends, pushing the liver and gallbladder toward your hand. Note findings. _____

_____

_____

NCLEX®-STYLE REVIEW QUESTIONS

Read each question carefully. Choose the best answer for each question.

1. The nurse is aware that the alimentary canal begins with what structure and ends where?
   1. Mouth and ends at the anus
   2. Esophagus and ends at the large intestine
   3. Jejunum and ends at the rectum
   4. Small intestine and ends at the large intestine

2. The nurse can refer to which of the following as accessory digestive organs? (Select all that apply.)
   1. Liver
   2. Pancreas
   3. Spleen
   4. Gallbladder
   5. Cecum

3. When performing a physical assessment on a client's abdomen, the nurse will follow which sequence of techniques?
   1. Inspection, palpation, percussion, auscultation
   2. Auscultation, inspection, palpation, percussion
   3. Auscultation, inspection, percussion, palpation
   4. Inspection, auscultation, percussion, palpation

4. When obtaining health history data from a pregnant female, the nurse must be sure to ask questions about what conditions? (Select all that apply.)
   1. Hemorrhoids
   2. Constipation
   3. Frequent voiding
   4. Nausea and vomiting
   5. Hernias

5. A 32-year-old male enters the medical clinic for an annual physical. He states that he has lost 22 lb in the last 2 months. What is an appropriate follow-up question from the nurse?
   1. "Was the weight loss intentional or unintentional?"
   2. "Did you join a fitness center?"
   3. "How much more weight do you want to lose?"
   4. "Good for you! Are you proud of yourself?"

6. Prior to starting the assessment of the abdomen, the nurse should do which of the following?
   1. Provide a warm, comfortable, and private environment
   2. Ask the client not to void for at least 1 hour
   3. Perform a pain assessment because the nurse should examine the painful area first
   4. Stand on the left side of the client

7. The nurse is caring for a second-day postoperative client following bowel surgery. The client has had a bowel movement or passed flatus since surgery. When the nurse auscultates the client's abdomen for bowel sounds, what would be an expected finding?
   1. Hyperactivity
   2. Normal
   3. Hypoactivity
   4. Borborygmi

8. The nurse begins percussion at the level of the umbilicus and moves toward the rib cage along the right midclavicular line. The percussion sounds change from tympany to dullness. What has the nurse identified?
   1. The lower border of the liver
   2. The lowest rib
   3. The spleen
   4. An abnormal finding

9. The nurse is about to palpate the abdomen of his client. The nurse should keep in mind that it is best to use which of the following techniques?
    1. Begin with a light palpation
    2. Slide his hand from each spot of the abdomen
    3. Use a bimanual technique for a cachexic client
    4. Use deep palpation if an abdominal aortic aneurysm is suspected

10. The nurse is aware that referred pain from the liver may be to what location?
    1. Left flank
    2. Right shoulder
    3. Jaw
    4. Right groin

22 Urinary System

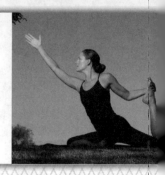

One may go a long way after one is tired.
—French Proverb

The elimination of waste products and toxins from the body is an important function of the urinary system. Without filtration by the kidneys, the accumulation of these products will affect the entire body. This chapter will focus on gathering both subjective and objective data related to the urinary system, as well as analysis of the data collected.

OBJECTIVES

At the completion of these exercises, you will be able to:

1. Review the anatomy and physiology of the urinary system.
2. Select the equipment necessary to complete the urinary assessment.
3. Identify the correct techniques for assessment of the urinary system.
4. Analyze subjective and objective data related to assessment of the urinary system.
5. Apply critical thinking in analysis of a case study.
6. Relate *Healthy People 2020* objectives to the assessment of the urinary system.
7. Assess the urinary system on a laboratory partner.
8. Document an assessment of the urinary system.
9. Complete NCLEX®-style review questions related to the urinary assessment.

ANATOMY & PHYSIOLOGY REVIEW

1. For each diagram below, label the structures as indicated by each line.

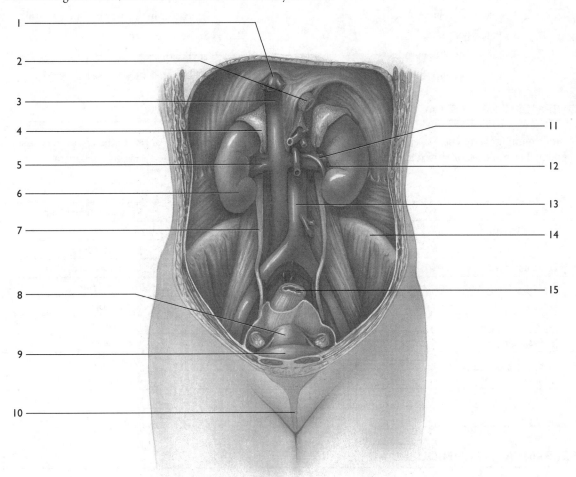

Anterior View of the Urinary Organs of a Female

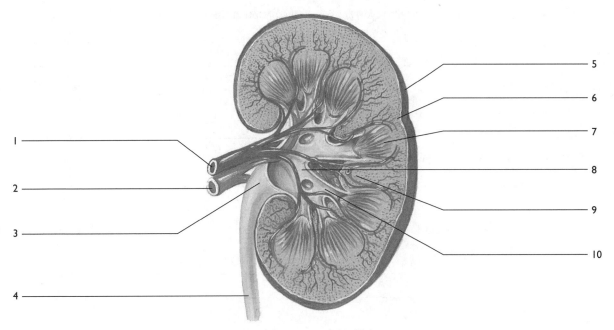

Internal Anatomy of the Kidney

2. Read each statement. Write a "K" on each line that relates to a function of the kidney or a "B" on each line that relates to the function of the bladder. Write "N/A" if it does not relate to the function of either organ.

_____ 1. Produces erythropoietin

_____ 2. Regulates volume of blood

_____ 3. Filters lymph

_____ 4. Eliminates waste products

_____ 5. Contracts during micturition

_____ 6. Temporarily stores urine

_____ 7. Assists in the metabolism of vitamin D

_____ 8. Secretes cortisol

_____ 9. Produces renin

_____ 10. Maintains acid–base balance

EQUIPMENT SELECTION

Prior to beginning the physical assessment of a client's urinary system, it is important to gather the appropriate assessment equipment. Place a check mark next to each piece of equipment that you would need to perform this assessment.

EQUIPMENT					
	Cotton balls		Lubricant		Sphygmomanometer
	Cotton-tipped applicator		Metric ruler		Stethoscope
	Culture media		Nasal speculum		Tape measure
	Dental mirror		Ophthalmoscope		Test tubes
	Doppler ultrasonic stethoscope		Otoscope		Thermometer
	Drape sheet		Penlight		Tongue blade
	Examination gown		Reflex hammer		Transilluminator
	Flashlight		Skinfold calipers		Tuning fork
	Gauze		Skin-marking pen		Vaginal speculum
	Gloves		Slides		Vision chart
	Goggles		Small towel		Watch with second hand
	Goniometer		Specimen containers		Wood's lamp

ASSESSMENT TECHNIQUES

Review each assessment technique. If the technique is correct, circle the number. If the technique is incorrect, write the correct assessment technique on the line provided.

1. The examiner should instruct the client to report any pain or discomfort during the assessment process.

_____

_____

2. Assessment of the urinary system should begin with the client sitting upright on an examination table with legs dangling.

_____

_____

3. The examiner should visually inspect the client's suprapubic area.

_____

_____

4. The bell of the stethoscope should be placed over each renal artery at the midclavicular line about 1 to 2 cm above the level of the umbilicus.

_____

_____

5. The costovertebral angles are inspected while the client is in a supine position.

_____

_____

6. Palpation over the costovertebral angles should initially be done with deep pressure.

_____

_____

7. Indirect percussion is used by placing the palm of the examiner's nondominant hand over the left or right costovertebral angle and using the ulnar surface of the dominant hand to thump the back of the nondominant hand.

_____

_____

8. The client should take and hold a deep breath throughout the entire capture maneuver of a kidney.

_____

_____

9. The fundus of the bladder can be located easily with light palpation.

_____

_____

10. Percussion of the bladder should begin over the suprapubic area and proceed superiorly toward the umbilicus.

_____

_____

ASSESSMENT FINDINGS

Read each assessment finding. Identify the finding as normal or abnormal by writing "N" for normal or "A" for abnormal on each line provided. In addition, identify each finding as either subjective or objective by writing "S" for subjective or "O" for objective on each line provided.

_____ **1.** Nonpalpable kidney

_____ **2.** Dark, cloudy urine

_____ **3.** Burning at time of voiding

_____ **4.** Oliguria

_____ **5.** Puffiness in the face

_____ **6.** CVA tenderness

_____ **7.** Pruritus of the skin

_____ **8.** Suprapubic tenderness

_____ **9.** Calculi

_____ **10.** Bladder distention

_____ **11.** Incontinence of urine

_____ **12.** Urethral discharge

_____ **13.** Palpable smooth, round, firm kidney

_____ **14.** Upper abdominal bruit in young adult

_____ **15.** Colic

_____ **16.** Hematuria

_____ **17.** Frequency

_____ **18.** Dry, scaly skin

_____ **19.** Urgency to void

_____ **20.** An elevation over the costovertebral angle

APPLICATION OF THE CRITICAL THINKING PROCESS

Read the scenario below and then answer the questions that follow in the space provided.

Romul is a 32-year-old male who is attending a family barbeque when he suddenly feels a sharp stabbing pain in his mid-back with a wave of nausea. The pain lasts approximately 20 min and resolves on its own. Unfortunately, 2 hours later the pain returns. It is more intense, and Romul begins to vomit. His brother becomes concerned and drives him to the emergency department.

Romul is 5′11″ and 325 lb. He has a history of a gastric bypass surgery 4 months ago. He has lost 42 lb since the surgery and has had no complications during his recovery. He does 30 minutes of cardiovascular activity every day and participates in a weight training class three times per week. He takes a multivitamin daily and two types of antihypertensive medication to regulate his blood pressure. As the nurse begins to interview Romul, she finds that he has only had an instant breakfast drink for breakfast and a plate of salad and barbequed chicken for lunch. The pain continues to intensify, and he rates it as a 12 on a scale of 0 to 10. He rolls over onto his side and begins to scream out in agony. He states his groin is starting to hurt him. When asked for a urine sample, gross hematuria is noted.

1. How should the nurse proceed with the physical assessment?

2. Should the nurse consider medicating the client for the severe pain prior to performing the physical assessment? Support your answer.

After a complete assessment including diagnostic testing, it is determined that Romul has a 6-mm renal calculus. (Additional resources may be needed to answer the following questions.)

3. What risk factors did Romul have for a renal calculus?

Romul will require lithotripsy (a medical procedure that uses shock waves to break up a calculus).

4. Write two priority nursing diagnoses for this client.

   1.

   2.

5. Romul and his family are concerned that this could happen to him again. The nurse prepares to educate Romul on the prevention of renal calculi. Develop a teaching plan for this scenario.

Goal:			
Objectives:	Content:	Teaching Strategies:	Evaluation:

HEALTHY PEOPLE 2020

Read the *Healthy People 2020* objective and answer the questions that follow in the space provided.

A *Healthy People 2020* objective is:

Reduce the rate of new cases of end-stage renal disease (ESRD).

1. What conditions increase a client's risk for developing ESRD?

2. Discuss how a nurse can use this objective to promote and maintain health and function of the urinary system.

ASSESSMENT AND DOCUMENTATION

Perform an assessment of the urinary system on your lab partner and document your findings on the following documentation form.

URINARY SYSTEM

Name:_____Date:_____

Age: _____ Gender: _____ Weight: _____

FOCUSED INTERVIEW

Reason for today's visit: _____

_____

General Questions

What are your normal patterns when you urinate? How often do you urinate each day? How much do you pass each time you urinate? _____

_____

_____

Have you noticed any change from your normal urination patterns? Have you noticed any changes in your pattern recently? Have you had any of these changes: urinating more often, urinating less often, urinating more fluid, or urinating less fluid? _____

_____

_____

When you urinate, do you feel you are able to empty your bladder completely? _____

_____

Are you always able to control when you are going to urinate? If not, do you have to hurry to the bathroom as soon as you feel the urge to urinate? When you feel the urge to urinate, are you able to get to the toilet? Have you ever had an "accident" and wet yourself? Have you ever urinated by accident when you have coughed, sneezed, or lifted a heavy object? _____

_____

_____

Do you ever have to get up at night to urinate? If so, can you describe why? Is there any predictable pattern? How many times per night? Describe your fluid intake for a day. _____

_____

_____

Do you have difficulty starting the flow of the stream? Does the stream flow continuously, or does it start and stop? Do you need to strain or push during urination to empty your bladder completely? _____

_____

_____

If you have urinary problems, have they caused you embarrassment or anxiety? Have your urinary problems affected your social, personal, or sexual relationships? _____

_____

_____

Has anyone is your family had a kidney disease or urinary problem? If so, when did they have it? How was it treated? Do they still have it? _____

_____

_____

Have you had a recent urine analysis or blood work evaluating your kidneys? If so, do you know the results?

_____

_____

Questions Related to Illness or Infection

Have you ever been diagnosed with a disease of the kidney or bladder? When were you diagnosed with the problem? What treatment was prescribed for the problem? Was the treatment helpful? What kinds of things do you do to help with the problem? Has the problem ever recurred (acute)? How are you managing the disease now (chronic)? _____

_____

_____

Do you now have or have you had an infection in the urinary system? When were you diagnosed with the infection? What treatment was prescribed for the problem? Was the treatment helpful? What kinds of things do you do to help with the problem? Has the problem ever recurred (acute)? How are you managing the infection now (chronic)? _____

_____

_____

Have you had surgery on the urinary system? If so, describe the procedure. How long ago did you have it done? Is the problem corrected? If not, describe it. Has anyone in your family ever had surgery on the urinary system? If so, please describe the procedure. How long ago was the surgery? Is the problem corrected? If not, describe it. _____

_____

_____

Do you have any of these problems: high blood pressure, diabetes, frequent bladder infections, kidney stones? If so, how has the problem been treated? Describe any associated symptoms. Do you still have problems with this condition? Do you have any idea what causes this problem? _____

_____

_____

Do you have any of these neurologic diseases: multiple sclerosis, Parkinson's disease, spinal cord injury, or stroke? If so, which one? When was it diagnosed? How are you being treated? _____

_____

_____

Do you have any type of cardiovascular disease? If so, what was the diagnosis? When was it diagnosed? How are you being treated? _____

_____

_____

Have you had influenza, a skin infection, a respiratory tract infection, or other infection recently? If so, what was it? What medication did the healthcare provider prescribe? Did you take all of the medication? Is this a recurrent problem? _____

_____

_____

Questions Related to Symptoms, Pain, and Behaviors

Symptoms

Have you noticed any changes in the quality of the urine? If so, describe the change. Has your urine been cloudy? Does it have an odor? Has the color changed? If there has been a color change, what is it? Does the color change happen each time you urinate? Is there a pattern? Can you predict the color change?

_____

_____

_____

If the urine is bloody (hematuria), the nurse should ask the following questions: Have you fallen recently? Do you experience burning when the blood is present? Have you seen clots in the urine? Have you noticed any stones or other material in the urine? Have you noticed any granular material on the toilet paper after you wipe? _____

_____

_____

Is your urine foamy and amber in color? _____

_____

Have you had any weight gain recently? If so, describe it. Are you retaining fluid? Are your rings, clothing, or shoes becoming tighter? Has this change been gradual or did it come on suddenly? _____

_____

Have you noticed any discharge from the urethra? If so, describe the color, odor, amount, and frequency. When did it start? Is this a recurrent problem? If so, what was the diagnosis? How was it treated? Did you follow the treatment as prescribed by the physician? _____

_____

Have you noticed any redness or other discoloration in the urethral area or penis? If so, describe the characteristics. _____

_____

For male clients: Do you have prostate problems? If so, describe the symptoms and treatment. When was your last prostate exam? _____

_____

Has your skin changed recently? Describe the change. Has the color changed? Is it itchy all the time? _____

_____

Have you recently had nausea, vomiting, diarrhea, or chills? If so, which one? Describe it. How was it treated? Has it recurred? _____

_____

Have you had any shortness of breath or difficulty breathing lately? If so, describe it. _____

_____

Do you have difficulty concentrating, reading, or remembering things? _____

_____

Pain

Do you ever have pain, burning, or other discomfort before, during, or after urination? If so, describe the discomfort, location, and timing. Do you have symptoms all of the time or some of the time? Is the discomfort predictable? Do you feel it after sexual intercourse? _____

_____

Do you have pain or discomfort in your back, sides, or abdomen? If so, show me where the pain or discomfort is located. Describe the pain. What aggravates or alleviates the symptoms? _____

_____

_____

Have you noticed any pain or discomfort when your urine is bloody? If so, describe the type, location, and timing of the discomfort. _____

_____

Behaviors

Describe your diet. What have you eaten and had to drink during the past week? How is your appetite? On a typical day, how much do you eat and drink? Do you drink alcoholic beverages? How many glasses of water do you drink a day? Are there any foods or beverages that bother you? Do any foods or beverages cause you discomfort either before or upon urination? Do any foods or beverages cause you to feel bloated or gassy? Do any foods or beverages alter the color, clarity, or smell of your urine? How much salt do you use?

Do you retain fluid after consuming certain foods or beverages? _____

_____

_____

_____

_____

Do you smoke or are you exposed to passive smoke? If so, what type of smoking (cigarette, cigar, pipe)? For how long? How many packs per day? _____

_____

_____

Do you use any recreational drugs? If so, describe the type, amount, and frequency. How long have you been using these drugs? _____

_____

How often do you have intercourse? Do you urinate after intercourse? Are you aware of any sexual partners who may have a sexually transmitted infection? _____

_____

_____

For female clients: How do you cleanse yourself after urination or a bowel movement? Do you use bubble bath? Do you use sprays, powders, or feminine hygiene products? _____

_____

_____

Age-Related Questions

Infants and Children

Have you ever been told that the child has a kidney that has failed to grow? _____

_____

Has the child ever been diagnosed with a kidney disorder? If so, what is it called, what were the symptoms, and how was it treated? Is it still being treated? _____

_____

Has the child had hearing problems? _____

Have you ever observed any unusual shape or structure in the child's genital anatomy? _____

_____

Has the child ever had problems with involuntary urination? If so, what are the characteristics? What was the diagnosis? How was it treated? Is it still occurring? _____

_____

Have you started toilet training with the child? If yes, how successful has it been? Are there any current problems with toilet training? What method are you using for toilet training? _____

_____

Has the child decreased play activity? _____

Are you changing the baby's diaper more or less than you were? _____

Pregnant Females

Have you noticed any changes in your urinary pattern? Have you noticed unusual swelling in your ankles, feet, fingers, or wrists? Have you noticed any headaches? _____

_____

_____

Older Adults

Have you noticed any unusual swelling in your ankles, feet, fingers, or wrists? _____

_____

For male clients: Have you noticed difficulty initiating the stream of urine, voiding in small amounts, and feeling the need to void more frequently than in the past? _____

_____

_____

Questions Related to the Environment

Internal Environment

What medications do you currently take? What medications have you been taking for the past several months? Describe the type, the dose, and the reason why you are taking the medication. How often do you take it? Every day, as needed, or only when you remember? _____

_____

_____

Do you take any vitamins, protein powders, or dietary supplements? If so, which ones? How much do you take? How many days a week do you take it? How many times a day? Why do you take it? _____

_____

_____

External Environment

Do you live in an environment or work in an industry that exposes you to toxic chemicals? _____

_____

Have you traveled recently to a foreign country or any unfamiliar place? _____

_____

PHYSICAL ASSESSMENT

General Survey

Position the client in a supine position with the abdomen exposed from the nipple line to the pubis. Assess the general appearance of the area: color, hydration status, scales, masses, indentations, or scars.

_____

_____

Inspect the abdomen for color, contour, symmetry, and distention. _____

_____

Auscultate the right and left renal arteries to assess circulatory sounds. _____

_____

For a client with a urinary catheter, inspect the catheter for signs of infection, correct placement, and urinary outflow. _____

_____

The Kidneys and Flanks

Position the client in a sitting position facing away from you. Inspect the left and right costovertebral angles, along with the flanks, for color and symmetry. _____

_____

If the client denies pain or discomfort in the pelvic region, the nurse may percuss and palpate. Gently palpate the area over the left costovertebral angle. Use blunt or indirect percussion to further assess the kidneys. Repeat the procedure on the right side. Ask the client to describe the sensation as you examine each side. _____

_____

_____

Advanced Skill: Palpating the Left and Right Kidney (Should not be attempted by novice nurses without supervision.)

The Urinary Bladder

Lightly palpate the bladder to determine symmetry, location, size, and sensation. _____

_____

_____

Percuss the bladder to determine its location and degree of fullness. _____

_____

NCLEX®-STYLE REVIEW QUESTIONS

Read each question carefully. Choose the best answer for each question.

1. The nurse understands that females are more likely than males to develop urinary tract infections for what reason?
   1. The length of the female urethra is longer than the male's
   2. The proximity of the urethral meatus to the rectum is closer in females
   3. Females are more likely to take bubble baths
   4. Females and males are equally as likely to develop a urinary tract infection

2. The nurse identifies the area of the lower back formed by the vertebral column and the downward curve of the last posterior rib as what area?
   1. Symphysis pubis
   2. Costovertebral angle
   3. Cortex
   4. Rectus abdominis

3. The nurse knows that formation of kidney stones can be attributed to conditions that increase the client's level of which electrolyte?
   1. Potassium
   2. Sodium
   3. Phosphorus
   4. Calcium

4. An older adult male presents to the emergency department complaining of blood in his urine. Which of the following questions would be appropriate for the nurse to include in assessing this client? (Select all that apply.)
   1. "Have you been passing any blood clots?"
   2. "Tell me about any recent falls."
   3. "Tell me about any pain you have had or may be having."
   4. "Do you take a multivitamin every day?"
   5. "Do you take aspirin every day?"

5. The nurse is beginning to assess the urinary system of a client. What is the best position in which to place the client?
   1. Prone
   2. Supine
   3. Lithotomy
   4. High-Fowler's

6. What would the nurse explain to a new graduate nurse about auscultation of the renal arteries for bruits?
   1. Auscultation is not necessary in the urinary assessment because it is performed during the abdominal assessment
   2. Auscultation is done by placing the bell of the stethoscope over the umbilical and epigastric areas
   3. Auscultation is performed last during the urinary assessment
   4. Auscultation is only necessary if the client complains of flank pain

7. The nurse identifies which of the following conditions as one that puts a client at higher risk for end-stage renal disease?
   1. Hypertension
   2. Obesity
   3. Frequent kidney infections
   4. Hydronephrosis

8. The nurse notes a distended bladder on physical assessment of a client. In describing this finding, the nurse uses which of the following terms?
   1. Tender and firm
   2. Smooth, round, and taut
   3. Boggy
   4. A distended bladder is not palpable

9. An older adult female complains of leaking urine whenever she coughs, sneezes, or laughs hard. What does the nurse document with this subjective finding?
   1. Total incontinence
   2. Functional incontinence
   3. Stress incontinence
   4. Reflex incontinence

10. When developing a teaching plan for a client who develops frequent renal calculi, the nurse should include which of the following?
    1. Drink enough fluids to produce 2,000 ml of urine per day
    2. Drink large amounts of caffeinated beverages
    3. Drink lots of milk
    4. Drink enough fluids to produce 4,800 ml of urine per day

23 Male Reproductive System

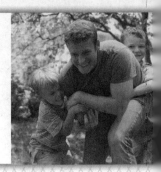

The difference between the impossible and the possible lies in a person's determination.
—Tommy Lasorda

The male reproductive system consists of multiple organs that are responsible for the production of hormones and male reproductive cells. The system has a great impact on male sexual behavior and requires a comprehensive assessment that includes psychosocial, self-care, and environmental factors. This chapter will focus on gathering both subjective and objective data related to the male reproductive system, as well as analysis of the data collected.

OBJECTIVES

At the completion of these exercises, you will be able to:

1. Review the anatomy and physiology of the male reproductive system.
2. Identify the correct techniques for assessment of the male reproductive system.
3. Analyze subjective and objective data related to assessment of the male reproductive system.
4. Recognize factors that can influence assessment findings.
5. Apply critical thinking in analysis of a case study.
6. Relate objectives in *Healthy People 2020* to the male reproductive system.
7. Assess the male reproductive system on a lab partner and an anatomic model.
8. Document an assessment of the male reproductive system.
9. Complete NCLEX®-style questions related to the assessment of the male reproductive system.

ANATOMY & PHYSIOLOGY REVIEW

1. For each of the following diagrams, label the structures as indicated by each line.

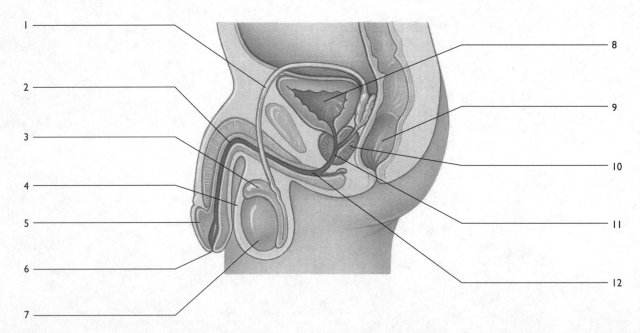

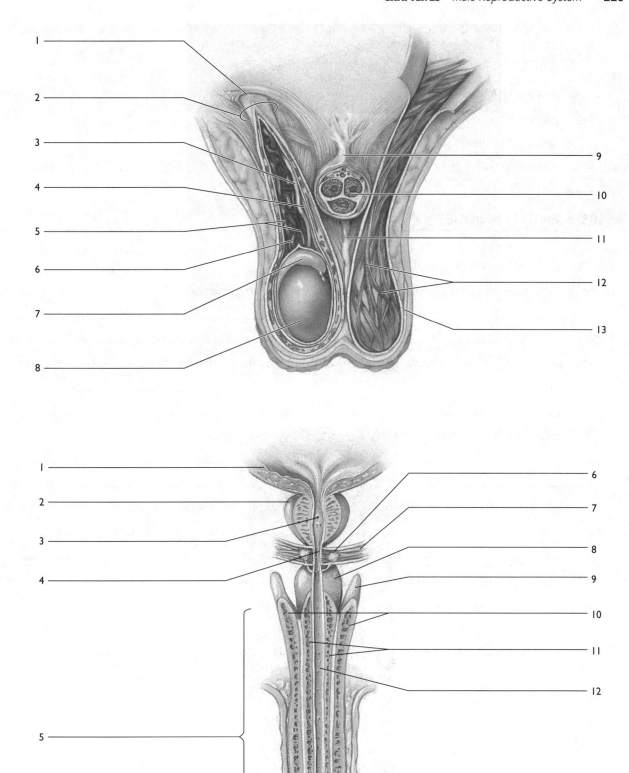

2. The following structures are part of the pathway for sperm. Place them in correct order from origin to ejaculation by placing numbers 1 to 6, where 1 represents the point of origin, on the line corresponding to the structure.

_____ Spermatic cord

_____ Ductus deferens

_____ Epididymis

_____ Seminiferous tubules

_____ Ejaculatory duct

_____ Seminal vesicles

ASSESSMENT TECHNIQUES

Review each assessment technique. If the technique is correct, circle the number. If the technique is incorrect, write the correct assessment technique on the line provided.

1. The client should be instructed to empty his bladder and bowel prior to the assessment.

_____

_____

2. Explain to the client that if an erection occurs during the assessment that this is normal and has no sexual connotation.

_____

_____

3. The client should be in the supine position for the first portion of this assessment.

_____

_____

4. If the client is uncircumcised, it is inappropriate for the examiner to ask the client to retract the foreskin.

_____

_____

5. Position of the urinary meatus should be assessed during the inspection of the penis.

_____

_____

6. To allow adequate visualization of the scrotum, the examiner should hold the penis firmly in the left hand and lift.

_____

_____

7. Transillumination of the scrotum can be performed by placing a lighted flashlight behind the scrotum in a well-lit room.

_____

_____

8. The client should breathe normally at first when the nurse is inspecting the right and left inguinal areas.

_____

_____

9. The finger pads should be used to palpate the anterior side of each testicle to locate the epididymis.

_____

_____

10. When palpating the bulbourethral gland, the examiner's index finger should gently be inserted into the anus with the thumb gently pressing against the perianal area. The examiner's index finger should gently press away from the thumb.

_____

_____

ASSESSMENT FINDINGS

Read each assessment finding. Identify the finding as normal or abnormal by writing an "N" for normal or an "A" for abnormal on each line provided.

_____ 1. Firm prostate

_____ 2. Heavy distribution of hair at the symphysis pubis on the adult

_____ 3. Smegma

_____ 4. Hard and beaded spermatic cord

_____ 5. Nonpalpable inguinal lymph nodes

_____ 6. Negative occult blood

_____ 7. Soft and boggy scrotal sac

_____ 8. Pinpoint-size meatus

_____ 9. Genital itching

_____ 10. Phimosis

_____ 11. Pain upon palpation of the bulbourethral gland

_____ 12. Prostate extends 1/2 cm into rectal area

_____ 13. Walnut-sized testis in an adult

_____ 14. A bulge at the external ring

_____ 15. Darker skin around the anus

_____ 16. Nits

_____ 17. Hypospadias

_____ 18. Decreased libido

_____ 19. Torsion of the testicle

_____ 20. Decreased ability to maintain an erection

FACTORS THAT INFLUENCE PHYSICAL ASSESSMENT FINDINGS

Fill in the blank(s) to complete each statement.

1. Cultural and religious beliefs may influence a family's decision to _____ a newborn male.

2. Dense pubic hair and penile and testicular enlargement in a male under the age of 10 is characterized as _____ _____.

3. Testicular cancer occurs more frequently in _____ than in any other ethnic group.

4. Drugs and alcohol may _____ a client's sexual drive.

5. During puberty, elevated _____ levels will cause the development of adult sexual characteristics.

6. The most common type of cancer in males between the ages of 20 and 35 is _____.

7. Cryptorchidism, also known as _____ testicles, is common in preterm male infants.

8. Diminished libido may occur in the older adult male because of a decreased level of _____.

9. Sexual interests and urges that are acted on prior to counseling of safe sex practices can put an adolescent at risk for _____ _____ _____.

10. Some signs of _____ _____ in male children may be depression, eating disorders, and swelling of the genitalia.

The Testicular Exam

Use the words in the Word Bank to complete each statement regarding the self-testicular exam.

Word Bank

monthly	cold	gentle pressure
shower	epididymis	firm
smooth	lumps	round
adolescence		

1. The self-testicular exam should be performed _____.

2. Males should begin doing self-testicular exams during _____.

3. Do not perform the self-testicular exam if your hands are _____.

4. The best time to perform the self-testicular exam is during a/an _____.

5. Feel each testicle by applying _____.

6. The contour of the testicle should be _____, _____, and _____.

7. You will feel the _____ on top of and behind each testicle.

8. The testicle should not have any _____.

APPLICATION OF THE CRITICAL THINKING PROCESS

Read each of the scenarios below and then answer the questions that follow in the space provided.

SCENARIO 1

Hugh is a 32-year-old male who is 5′9″ tall and weighs 250 lb. He is the author of several best-selling novels and spends a great deal of time using his laptop. He has been riding his bike 10 to 15 miles per day in order to lose some weight. He began having a constant pain in his rectal area 4 days ago. He assumed the pain was from the bicycle seat being hard and the bounce from some of his trail rides. Today he is being seen in the clinic for "pain in the rectal area." He states the pain is "very sharp and so bad he can barely sit down"; he prefers to stand during the interview. The pain is now a 7 on a scale of 0 to 10. He admits to sitting in a hot bath and taking Tylenol for the pain, which has resulted in minimal relief.

The physical assessment yields the following information: BP 130/82, P 104, RR 20, T 100.7. His general skin color is pale. In the sacrococcygeal area, there is dimpling noted with erythema, moderate edema, and warmth to the area. In the center of the dimpling, a small coarse hair is noted with a small amount of yellow, foul-smelling drainage.

1. Using the information in the scenario, complete the OLDCART & ICE pain assessment.

O

L

D

C

A

R

T

I

C

E

2. Are additional questions needed to complete the pain assessment? Explain.

3. List three focused questions related to sexuality that may be asked.

1. _____

2. _____

3. _____

4. The nurse suspects that Hugh has a pilonidal cyst. What data support this suspicion?

5. The client asks the nurse "How did this happen, and how can I make sure this doesn't happen again?" The nurse explains the risk factors for developing a pilonidal cyst as (additional resources may be needed to answer this question):

The nurse reports her findings to the doctor. She assists him in an incision and drainage (I&D) procedure to clean out the infected wound. The doctor then sends the client home with a dressing and a prescription for an antibiotic and analgesic. The client returns to the clinic in 5 days. He states "I have no pain; I feel so much better!" His vital signs are BP 110/62, HR 72, RR 12, Temp 97.8°. During inspection of the wound there is a mild amount of erythema at the incision and no edema or drainage present.

6. Document an APIE note using the information provided in the scenario.

A

P

I

E

SCENARIO 2

Felix is a 73-year-old male being examined in the clinic for testicular discomfort. He has been widowed for 10 years and has never had any children. He was told he was infertile when he was 28 years old after trying to have children with his wife for almost 5 years. His doctor told him his infertility was probably related to his history of cryptorchidism as an infant. The nurse is gathering subjective data.

1. List three focused questions the nurse should ask this client.

1.

2.

3.

2. Felix is uncircumcised. Discuss additional measures that must be taken during the assessment of the penis of an uncircumcised male.

3. Upon completion of the physical assessment, the healthcare provider discusses the findings with the nurse and states, "The finding of a large palpable mass is suggestive of testicular cancer." List two risk factors for testicular cancer that may be revealed in a health history.

    1.

    2.

4. Transillumination of the scrotum is performed. Describe the anticipated findings of transillumination of the scrotum when a mass is present.

HEALTHY PEOPLE 2020

Read the *Healthy People 2020* objective and answering the questions that follow in the space provided.

A *Healthy People 2020* objective is:

Reduce gonorrhea rates.

1. List four signs or symptoms of gonorrhea.

    1. _____

    2. _____

    3. _____

    4. _____

2. Discuss how a nurse on a college campus can use this objective to promote and maintain the health of the students.

ASSESSMENT AND DOCUMENTATION

Perform an assessment of the male reproductive system. Complete the subjective data collection on a lab partner (answers may be fabricated) and complete the objective data collection on an anatomical model. Document your findings on the following documentation form.

MALE REPRODUCTIVE SYSTEM

Name:_____Date:_____

Age: _____ Sexual Preference: _____

FOCUSED INTERVIEW

Reason for today's visit: _____

_____

General Questions

Are you sexually active?

    If no, explain why: _____

If yes, answer the following:

    Frequency: _____

    Number of current partners: _____

    Number of partners in the past: _____

    Type of sexual activities: _____

    Type of contraceptive used: _____

    Safe sex practices: _____

    Do you have any difficulties becoming aroused? _____

    Are you able to achieve and maintain an erection? _____

    Use of erectile enhancers: _____

    Use of lubricants/devices/other enhancers: _____

During an erection, is the shaft of the penis straight or crooked? _____

Are you able to achieve orgasm? _____

Discuss your satisfaction with your sexual habits: _____

_____

Describe any changes in your sex drive in the past:

    Month: _____

    Year: _____

Are you able to talk to your partner about your sexual needs? _____

Do your family and friends support your relationship with your sexual partner? _____

Have you ever been in a relationship that you found to be sexually abusive? _____

Have you ever tried to have children? _____

Have you ever sought help for fertility issues? _____

Current medical conditions: _____

Past surgeries: _____

Have you been circumcised? _____

Medication (prescribed, over the counter, home remedies, herbal or cultural medicines, or dietary supplements): _____

Tobacco use: _____

Alcohol use: _____

Recreational drug use: _____

Hepatitis immunization: _____

Do you perform testicular self-examinations? _____

Have you ever been diagnosed with a sexually transmitted infection? _____

Have you ever had intercourse with someone who has been diagnosed with a sexually transmitted infection? _____

Have you ever been tested for a sexually transmitted infection? _____

Are you aware of any exposure to HIV? _____

Are you aware of any exposure to hepatitis? _____

Describe any exposure to lead, chemicals, or toxins in the environment: _____

Describe the use of any protective equipment when engaged in work or athletic activities: _____

Age-Related Questions

Infants and Children

Redness, swelling, or discharge that is discolored or foul smelling in the child's genital area: _____

Asymmetry, lumps, or masses in the infant's genitals: _____

Any complaints of itching, burning, or swelling in the genital area? _____

The nurse should ask older children the following:

Has anyone ever touched you when you didn't want him or her to? _____

Has anyone ever asked you to touch him or her when you didn't want to? _____

Where did he or she ask you to touch him or her? _____

Who touched you? _____ How many times did this happen? _____ Who knows about this? _____

Adolescents

Reinforce confidentiality while educating about teen pregnancy, birth control, and protection against sexually transmitted infections.

Vaccinations (Gardasil): _____

Older Adults

Have you perceived any changes in your sexuality related to advanced age? _____

Symptoms or Behaviors

Do you now or have you ever had:

Lumps or masses:

Penis: _____

Scrotum: _____

Surrounding areas: _____

Swelling:

Penis: _____

Scrotum: _____

Surrounding areas: _____

Pain:

    Penis: _____

    Scrotum: _____

    Surrounding areas: _____

    Discharge: _____

    Color changes: _____

    Itching: _____

Rectum:

    Pain: _____

    Itching: _____

    Burning: _____

    Bleeding: _____

    Incontinence: _____

PHYSICAL ASSESSMENT

Vital signs: _____ BP _____ HR _____ RR _____ Temp

Inspection

Pubic hair:

    Distribution: _____

    Amount: _____

    Texture: _____

    Hygiene: _____

Penis:

    Size: _____

    Pigmentation: _____

    Venous pattern: _____

    Lesions: _____

    Smegma: _____

    Foreskin: _____

    Urinary meatus: _____

Scrotum:

    Shape: Right: _____   Left: _____

    Pigmentation: Right: _____   Left: _____

    Veins: Right: _____   Left: _____

    Lesions: Right: _____   Left: _____

    Swelling: Right: _____   Left: _____

Perianal area:

    Pigmentation: _____

    Swelling: _____

    Lesions: _____

Palpation

Penis:

    Texture: _____

    Meatus: _____

    Tenderness: _____

    Lumps/nodules: _____

Scrotum:

    Texture: Right: _____   Left: _____

    Tenderness: Right: _____   Left: _____

    Lumps/nodules: Right: _____   Left: _____

    Testes:

        Texture: Right: _____   Left: _____

        Shape: Right: _____   Left: _____

        Tenderness: Right: _____   Left: _____

    Epididymis:

        Shape: Right: _____   Left: _____

        Tenderness: Right: _____   Left: _____

    Spermatic cord: _____

Inguinal region:

    Femoral artery: Right: _____   Left: _____

    Lymph nodes: Right: _____   Left: _____

    Swelling: Right: _____   Left: _____

    Tenderness: Right: _____   Left: _____

    Hernias/bulges: Right: _____   Left: _____

Perianal area:

    Tenderness: _____

    Lumps/nodules: _____

    Anus: _____

    Bulbourethral gland: _____

    Prostate gland: _____

    External hemorrhoids: _____

NCLEX®-STYLE REVIEW QUESTIONS

Read each question carefully. Choose the best answer for each question.

1. Which of the following statements is true about the scrotum?
    1. The right side extends lower than the left
    2. The temperature is about 3 degrees warmer than core temperature
    3. A vertical septum divides it into two sections
    4. It is housed by the testes

2. Upon inspection of the newborn male's penis, which of the following would require further investigation?
    1. A hypospadias
    2. A penis size of 2.7 cm
    3. A scrotum that seems oversized
    4. Undescended testicles

3. During a focused interview, the nurse asks the client if he is aware if his mother received diethylstilbestrol (DES) treatment during pregnancy. This is important because sons who are born to mothers who have had DES are at higher risk for: (Select all that apply.)
    1. testicular cancer
    2. low sperm counts
    3. hypospadias
    4. cryptorchidism
    5. polycystic kidney disease

4. A 78-year-old male presents to the medical clinic with multiple questions about his fertility. He has recently married a 42-year-old female, and together they would like to have a child. The nurse must consider which of these age-related changes when discussing the possibility of reproduction with the client?
    1. The older male may produce viable sperm throughout his entire life span
    2. Sexual libido increases with age
    3. Older men who are on multiple types of medication should not try to attempt to reproduce
    4. Ejaculation in the older adult male does not change throughout the life span

5. A 41-year-old male presents to the medical clinic complaining of difficulty achieving an erection. Which of the following focused interview questions would be appropriate for the nurse to ask? (Select all that apply.)
    1. "Do you have a history of genitourinary surgery?"
    2. "What medications are you taking?"
    3. "Were you born with undescended testicles?"
    4. "At what age did you begin having sexual intercourse?"
    5. "Did you have chicken pox as a child?"

6. The best position for the male client to be in at the beginning of the physical assessment of the male reproductive structures is:
    1. supine
    2. semi-Fowler's
    3. standing upright
    4. left side-lying

7. During inspection of the male genitalia, the nurse notices small bluish-gray spots at the base of the pubic hairs. This finding can be indicative of:
    1. crab or pubic lice
    2. cryptorchidism
    3. smegma
    4. syphilitic lesions

8. The cremasteric reflex can occur in which type of an environment?
    1. Cold
    2. Hot
    3. Moist
    4. Stressful

9. Which instruction by the nurse is most appropriate to give a client while assessing for an inguinal hernia?
   1. "Cough or bear down."
   2. "Take a deep breath in."
   3. "Stand on one leg."
   4. "Bend over at the waist."

10. A 17-year-old lacrosse player suddenly develops severe unilateral testicular pain. His mother brings him to the pediatrician's office for an evaluation. Upon the initial assessment, the nurse suspects a testicular torsion. The nurse's next step should be to:
    1. inform the client that the healthcare provider is running behind and it may be about a 30-minute wait
    2. apply ice to the scrotum for 20 minutes while the client waits
    3. administer an analgesic because a torsion can be extremely painful
    4. call for the healthcare provider because the client might require immediate surgical intervention

24 Female Reproductive System

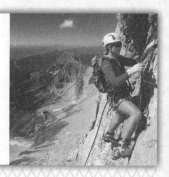

Our greatest glory is not in never failing, but in rising up every time we fail.
—Ralph Waldo Emerson

The female reproductive system consists of multiple organs that are responsible for the production of hormones and female reproductive cells. The system has a great impact on sexual behavior and requires a comprehensive assessment that will include psychosocial, self-care, and environmental factors. This chapter will focus on gathering both subjective and objective data related to the female reproductive system, as well as analysis of the data collected.

OBJECTIVES

At the completion of these exercises, you will be able to:

1. Review the anatomy and physiology of the female reproductive system.
2. Identify the correct techniques for assessment of the female reproductive system.
3. Analyze subjective and objective data related to assessment of the female reproductive system.
4. Recognize factors that can influence assessment findings.
5. Apply critical thinking in analysis of a case study.
6. Relate *Healthy People 2020* objectives to the female reproductive system.
7. Assess the female reproductive system on a model.
8. Document an assessment of the female reproductive system.
9. Complete NCLEX®-style review questions related to the assessment of the female reproductive system.

ANATOMY & PHYSIOLOGY REVIEW

1. For each of the following diagrams, label the structures as indicated by each line.

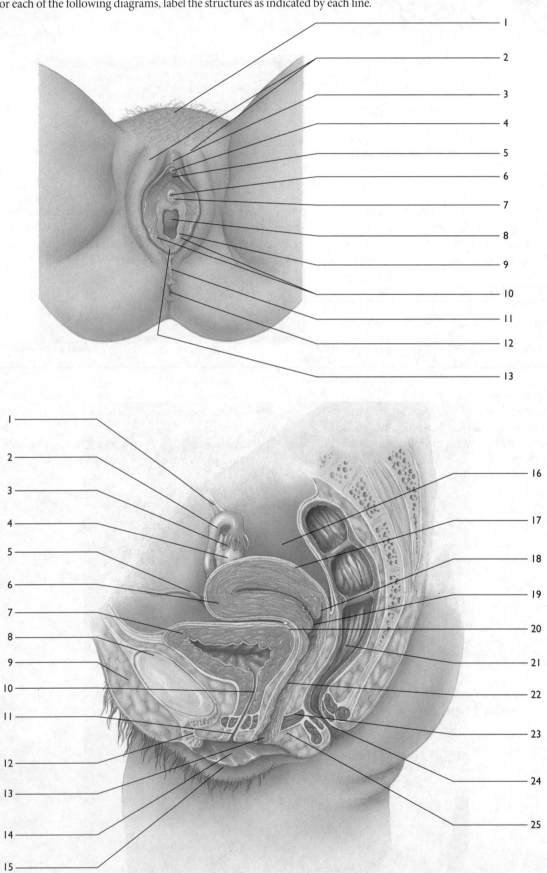

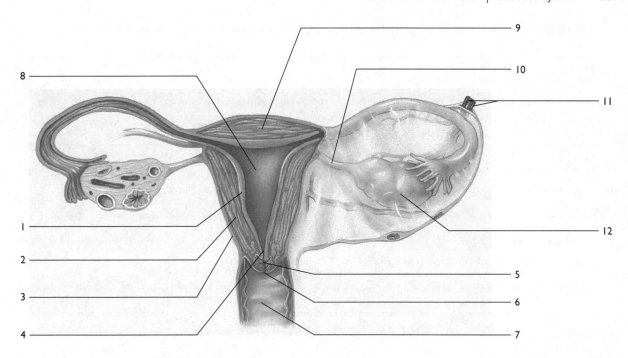

2. Circle the organ associated with each descriptor.

1.	Channel for menstrual flow	**Uterus**	**Vagina**	**Fallopian tubes**
2.	Produce ova	**Ovaries**	**Bartholin's glands**	**Fallopian tubes**
3.	The "birth canal"	**Fallopian tubes**	**Mons pubis**	**Vagina**
4.	Produce estrogen	**Ovaries**	**Skene's glands**	**Bartholin's glands**
5.	Produce(s) vaginal lubricant	**Vagina**	**Skene's glands**	**Bartholin's glands**
6.	Site of fertilization of the ovum	**Fallopian tubes**	**Ovaries**	**Uterus**
7.	Produce progesterone	**Ovaries**	**Skene's glands**	**Bartholin's glands**
8.	Protective sac for fetus	**Ovaries**	**Uterus**	**Introitus**
9.	Site of implantation of fertilized ovum	**Ovaries**	**Fallopian tubes**	**Uterus**
10.	Primary organ of sexual stimulation	**Introitus**	**Clitoris**	**Vagina**

ASSESSMENT TECHNIQUES

Review each assessment technique. If the technique is correct, circle the number. If the technique is incorrect, write the correct assessment technique on the line provided.

1. The client should be placed in the lithotomy position for the female reproductive assessment.

_____

_____

2. The hand of the nurse should separate the labia majora in order to inspect the clitoris and the urethral orifice.

_____

_____

3. The nurse should ask the client to bear down in order to inspect for any protrusions from the vagina.

_____

_____

4. When palpating the vaginal walls, the nurse should begin with the right palm facing down toward the floor.

_____

_____

5. When palpating for the Skene's glands, the nurse's right index finger should apply gentle pressure downward against the vaginal wall and a stroking movement should milk the gland.

_____

_____

6. Prior to insertion, the vaginal speculum should be placed in the nurse's nondominant hand.

_____

_____

7. A closed vaginal speculum should be inserted slowly at a 45-degree angle.

_____

_____

8. A slide or specimen container should be labeled and ready for specimen collection during the vaginal exam.

_____

_____

9. The nurse should remain seated during bimanual palpation.

_____

_____

10. The nurse should insert one finger into the vagina and one finger into the rectum to perform the rectovaginal exam.

_____

_____

ASSESSMENT FINDINGS

Read each assessment finding. Identify the finding as normal or abnormal by writing an "N" for normal or an "A" for abnormal on each line provided.

_____ 1. Moist, dark anus

_____ 2. Heavy distribution of hair at the mons pubis and sparse at the labia

_____ 3. Pink introitus

_____ 4. 30-day menstrual cycle

_____ 5. Discharge from Skene's gland

_____ 6. 1-cm long clitoris

_____ 7. Cervical polyp

_____ 8. Uterus slightly tilted upward

_____ 9. Genital itching

_____ 10. Nontender uterine wall

_____ 11. Pain upon palpation of Bartholin's glands

_____ 12. Firm perineum

_____ 13. Cystocele

_____ 14. Smooth and pink labia minora

_____ 15. Pink, moist cervix

_____ 16. Bluish-gray spots at the base of pubic hair

_____ 17. Clear vaginal discharge

_____ 18. Decreased libido

_____ 19. Nonpalpable ovary

_____ 20. Candidiasis

FACTORS THAT INFLUENCE PHYSICAL ASSESSMENT FINDINGS

Fill in the blank(s) to complete each statement.

1. Female genital mutilation is a cultural practice in _____, _____, and _____ countries.

2. The uterine capacity of a pregnant female can increase to _____ liters.

3. The female child reaches puberty _____ the male child.

4. Lesbian experimentation is developmentally _____ in adolescents.

5. The observed/palpated softening of the cervix during pregnancy is called _____ _____.

6. Human papillomavirus (HPV) increases a female's risk for _____ cancer.

7. Many religions forbid _____ _____.

8. Hydrocarbon polychlorinated biphenyls (PCBs) found in _____ manufacturing are associated with low birth weight, spontaneous abortion, hyperpigmentation of infants, and microcephaly.

9. Human papillomavirus quadrivalent (Gardasil) is a/an _____ that may protect females against most cervical cancers.

10. Nurses working in _____ and exposed to antineoplastic drugs may have a higher risk of irregular menstrual cycles and spontaneous abortions.

APPLICATION OF THE CRITICAL THINKING PROCESS

Read the scenario below and then answer the questions that follow in the space provided.

Shannon is a 23-year-old female college student. During a health and wellness fair on campus, she stopped at a booth set up by students in the nursing department to provide information about human papillomavirus (HPV). The booth was very crowded but Shannon was very anxious to learn if she was at risk for this virus.

1. List three focused questions that the student nurse should ask Shannon to assess her risk factors for HPV.

    1. _____
    2. _____
    3. _____

2. Shannon feels that she is at risk for HPV after speaking with a nursing student. She is now worried about how she can go about finding out if she has it. The nursing student explains that the HPV screening includes:

3. Shannon asks the nursing student where she could find out more information on HPV. The nursing student provides various resources to learn more.

    1. Name one campus resource:

    2. Name one website (provide address):

    3. Name one community-based (off-campus) resource:

4. Shannon decides to make an appointment with a women's health practitioner on her campus. What signs and symptoms may be noted during the physical assessment that would support the presence of HPV?

HEALTHY PEOPLE 2020

Read the *Healthy People 2020* objective and answer the questions that follow in the space provided.

A *Healthy People 2020* objective is:

Reduce the proportion of females ages 15 to 44 years who have ever required treatment for pelvic inflammatory disease (PID).

1. List four signs and symptoms of PID.

    1. _____
    2. _____
    3. _____
    4. _____

2. Discuss how a nurse at a women's health clinic can use this objective to promote and maintain health of the clients.

ASSESSMENT AND DOCUMENTATION

Perform an assessment of the female reproductive system. Complete the subjective data collection on a lab partner (answers may be fabricated) and complete the objective data collection on an anatomic model. Document your findings on the following documentation form.

FEMALE REPRODUCTIVE SYSTEM

Name:_____ Date:_____

Age: _____ Sexual Preference: _____

FOCUSED INTERVIEW

Reason for today's visit: _____

_____

General Questions

Do you have any concerns about your reproductive health? _____

_____

Current medical conditions: _____

Past surgeries: _____

Medication: _____

Hormonal therapy: _____

Tobacco use: _____

Alcohol use: _____

Recreational drug use: _____

Family history of female reproductive disease/disorders: _____

Describe any exposure to lead, chemicals, or toxins in the environment: _____

Menses:

How old were you when you had your first menses? _____

When was the first day of your last menstrual period? _____

How many days does your cycle last? _____

How many days does bleeding occur? _____

Describe your menstrual flow: _____

How do you usually feel during your period? _____

What type of feminine hygiene products do you use during your period? _____

_____

Do you take any medications to relieve symptoms during your period? _____

_____

Menopause:

When did menopause begin for you? _____

Tell me about physical changes you have noticed since menopause. _____

Have you had any vaginal bleeding since starting menopause? _____

Have you taken any medications or natural substances for menopausal symptoms? No _____

Yes _____ Explain _____

Age-Related Questions

Infants and Children

Have you noticed any redness, swelling, or discharge that is discolored or foul smelling in the child's genital area? _____

Has the child complained of itching, burning, or swelling in the genital area? _____

The nurse should ask the preschool- or school-age child the following questions:

Has anyone ever touched you when you didn't want him or her to?

Where? (*The nurse may want to have the child point to a picture or doll.*)

Has anyone ever asked you to touch him or her when you didn't want to?

Where did he or she ask you to touch him or her?

If the child answers "yes," the child may be experiencing sexual abuse. The nurse should try to obtain additional information by asking the following questions, but must remember to be sensitive:

Who touched you?

How many times did this happen?

Who knows about this?

Adolescents

Are you having sex with anyone? _____

Have you been taught that sexual intercourse can lead to pregnancy? _____

Do you understand that sexual intercourse can lead to sexually transmitted infections? _____

Pregnancy

Have you ever been pregnant? If so, how many times? _____

Do you have any children? _____

Have you had any miscarriages (spontaneous abortions) or induced abortions? _____

Describe any fertility problems you have experienced: _____

_____

Describe any difficulties you experienced during pregnancy: _____

Sexual Activity and Health History

Are you sexually active? _____

If no, explain why: _____

If yes, answer the following: _____

   Frequency: _____

   Number of current partners: _____

   Number of partners in the past: _____

   Type of sexual activities: _____

   Type of contraceptive used: _____

   Safe sex practices: _____

Do you have any difficulties becoming aroused? _____

Are you able to achieve sexual satisfaction? _____

Use of lubricants/devices/other enhancers: _____

Discuss your satisfaction or dissatisfaction with your sexual habits: _____

_____

Describe any changes in your sex drive in the past:

   Month: _____

   Year: _____

Are you able to talk to your partner about your sexual needs? _____

Do your family and friends support your relationship with your sexual partner?

_____

Have you ever been in a relationship that you found to be sexually abusive?

_____

Hepatitis immunization: _____

When was your last pap smear? Results? _____

Describe your hygiene practices: _____

Have you ever been tested for a sexually transmitted infection? _____

Have you ever been diagnosed with a sexually transmitted infection? _____

Have you ever had intercourse with someone who has been diagnosed with a sexually transmitted infection? _____

Are you aware of any exposure to HIV or hepatitis? _____

Symptoms or Behaviors

Genitalia

Do you now or have you ever had:

    Rashes: _____

    Blisters: _____

    Ulcers/sores: _____

    Warts: _____

    Lumps/masses: _____

    Swelling: _____

    Redness: _____

    Itching: _____

    Discharge: _____

    Bleeding: _____

    Odor: _____

    Pain: _____

    Rectum:

        Pain: _____

        Itching: _____

        Burning: _____

        Bleeding: _____

        Incontinence: _____

PHYSICAL ASSESSMENT

Vital signs: _____ BP _____ HR _____ RR _____ Temp

Inspection (on anatomic model)

Genitalia:

    Hair distribution: _____

    Amount: _____

    Texture: _____

    Hygiene: _____

    Skin color: _____

Labia majora:

    Symmetry: _____

    Color: _____

    Lesions: _____

    Texture: _____

    Integrity: _____

Labia minora:

    Symmetry: _____

    Color: _____

    Lesions: _____

    Texture: _____

    Integrity: _____

Clitoris:

    Midline: _____

    Texture: _____

    Color: _____

    Integrity: _____

Urethral orifice:

    Midline: _____

    Texture: _____

    Color: _____

    Integrity: _____

    Urine leakage: _____

Perineum:

    Texture: _____

    Color: _____

    Integrity: _____

    Lesions: _____

Palpation

Vaginal walls: _____

Urethra: _____

Skene's glands: _____

Bartholin's glands: _____

NCLEX®-STYLE REVIEW QUESTIONS

Read each question carefully. Choose the best answer for each question.

1. The nurse uses the word *introitus* to identify the:
   1. clitoris
   2. vaginal opening
   3. perineum
   4. cervix

2. The menstrual cycle is:
   1. defined by the first day of one period until the first day of the next
   2. defined by the last day of one period until the first day of the next
   3. defined by the first day of a period until the last day of the same period
   4. 28 days long

3. A 31-year-old female presents to the women's health clinic complaining of premenstrual syndrome (PMS). The nurse conducts a focused interview to gather more data. Which of the following symptoms would be expected during PMS?
   1. Weight loss
   2. A relaxed feeling
   3. Breast engorgement
   4. Nipple discharge

4. When preparing a client for the assessment of the female reproductive system, what is important for the nurse to explain to the client?
   1. What will happen during the exam
   2. The exam may be painful
   3. The nurse will conduct the exam as quickly as possible
   4. It is best to have a full bladder during the exam

5. During a pelvic examination, the nurse notes a client has raised, moist, cauliflower-shaped lesions on the labia majora. What diagnosis does the nurse anticipate?
   1. Normal finding
   2. Yeast infection
   3. Genital warts
   4. Pubic lice

6. The nurse identifies a young female client with sparse, dark, visibly pigmented, curly pubic hair on the labia as in which Tanner's stage of maturation?
   1. 2
   2. 3
   3. 4
   4. 5

7. When preparing to perform the speculum examination in a female client, what is the nurse's best action?
   1. Prewarm the speculum with warm water
   2. Lubricate the speculum with petroleum jelly
   3. Use the appropriate-sized speculum for the size of the client
   4. Hold the speculum in the nondominant hand

8. A 19-year-old female recently went for her annual gynecologic examination. During the examination the physician mentioned briefly that her uterus is retroverted. When the physician left the room, she immediately asked the nurse if this is something she should be worried about. What is the nurse's best response?
   1. The uterus is tilted forward and can be a normal variation
   2. The uterus is tilted backward and can be a normal variation
   3. The uterus is parallel to the tailbone and can cause difficulty during childbirth
   4. The uterus is tilted backward and can cause difficulty during childbirth

9. To obtain a gonorrhea culture, what is the most appropriate specimen collection technique?
   1. Insert a saline-moistened cotton applicator into the cervical os
   2. Insert the paddle end of a spatula into the fornix and rotate
   3. Insert a dry cotton applicator into the cervical os and leave in place for 1 full minute
   4. Insert a saline-moistened cotton applicator into the fornix

10. A 21-year-old female has been experiencing lower back pain and pelvic pain for 3 days. After careful examination, a small ovarian cyst is found. What is the nurse's best explanation for this client?
    1. She will need to have immediate surgery before it ruptures
    2. These fluid-filled vesicles are not cancerous
    3. This most likely will lead to ovarian cancer
    4. Ovarian cysts are common in females with sexually transmitted infections

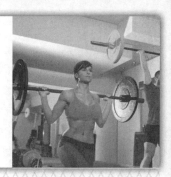

The way I see it, you can either run from it, or learn from it.
—Rafiki to Simba, *The Lion King*

Enjoying a quality life may depend on a client's ability to participate in routine and daily activities. Muscles, bones, and joints must all be functioning properly for the human body to move. Throughout the life span, many changes occur in the musculoskeletal system. This chapter will focus on gathering both subjective and objective data related to the musculoskeletal system, as well as analysis of the data collected.

OBJECTIVES

At the completion of these exercises, you will be able to:

1. Review the anatomy and physiology of the musculoskeletal system.
2. Identify the correct techniques for assessment of the musculoskeletal system.
3. Analyze subjective and objective data related to assessment of the musculoskeletal system.
4. Recognize factors that can influence assessment findings.
5. Apply critical thinking in analysis of a case study.
6. Relate *Healthy People 2020* objectives to the musculoskeletal system.
7. Assess the musculoskeletal system on a laboratory partner.
8. Document an assessment of the musculoskeletal system.
9. Complete NCLEX®-style review questions related to the assessment of the musculoskeletal system.

ANATOMY & PHYSIOLOGY REVIEW

1. For each of the following diagrams, label the structures as indicated by each line.

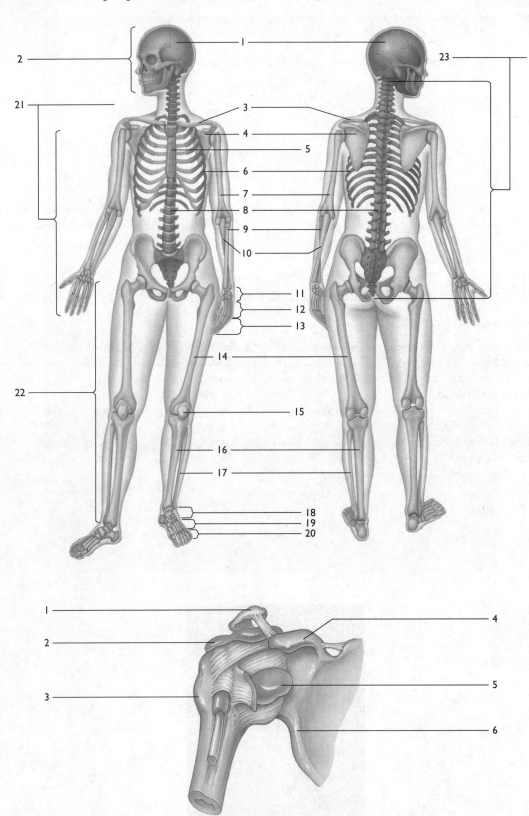

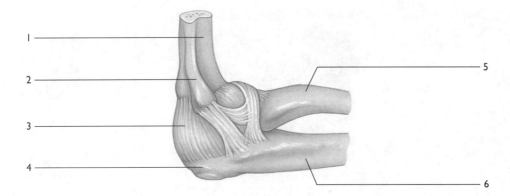

2. Read each statement, follow the instructions, and place the action on the diagram provided.

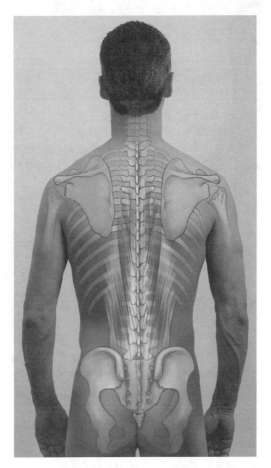

1. Connect the left iliac crest to the right iliac crest.

2. Connect the spinous process T_1 to the right posterior superior iliac spine.

3. Connect the spinous process C_7 to the left posterior superior iliac spine.

4. Draw a line between L_5 and S_1.

5. Circle the coccyx bone.

3. For each picture below, list the type of movement that is being displayed.

1. _____
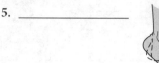
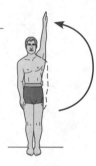

5. _____
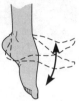
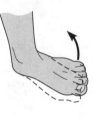

2. _____
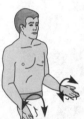

6. _____
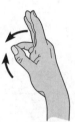

3. _____
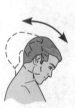

7. _____

4. _____

8. _____
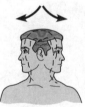
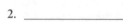

4. Circle the movements that each of the following joints is capable of performing.

1. Shoulder	Abduction	External rotation	Hyperextension
2. Wrist	Flexion	Supination	Radial deviation
3. Hip	Extension	Internal rotation	Pronation
4. Knee	Pronation	Extension	Hyperextension
5. Elbow	Supination	Flexion	Circumduction
6. Thumb	Radial deviation	Extension	Opposition
7. Ankle	Plantar flexion	Eversion	Lateral flexion
8. Spine	Rotation	Supination	Lateral flexion
9. Toe	Abduction	Adduction	Inversion
10. Finger	Circumduction	External rotation	Extension

ASSESSMENT TECHNIQUES

Review each assessment technique. If the technique is correct, circle the number. If the technique is incorrect, write the correct assessment technique on the line provided.

1. The index and middle fingers of the nurse should be positioned in front of the tragus when palpating the client's temporo-mandibular joint.

   _____

   _____

2. When assessing internal rotation of the shoulders, the nurse should ask the client to clasp his or her hands behind the head.

   _____

   _____

3. Abduction at the shoulder should be 50 degrees as demonstrated by extension of the arm.

   _____

   _____

4. When assessing for muscle strength, the nurse should provide opposing force while the client puts a joint through its range of motion.

   _____

   _____

5. To palpate the olecranon process, the nurse must palpate the junction between the acromion and the clavicle.

   _____

   _____

6. Auscultation is not a technique used in the musculoskeletal assessment.

   _____

   _____

7. During Phalen's test, the client's wrists should be bent with hands palm to palm.

   _____

   _____

8. Light percussion over the median nerve is used to assess Tinel's sign.

   _____

   _____

9. Range of motion of the spine begins with the neck.

   _____

   _____

10. Hyperextension of the spine should never be attempted.

   _____

   _____

ASSESSMENT FINDINGS

Read each assessment finding. Identify the finding as normal or abnormal by writing an "N" for normal or an "A" for abnormal on each line provided.

_____ 1. Symmetrical joints
_____ 2. Crepitus
_____ 3. Muscle Strength 1
_____ 4. Ganglion
_____ 5. Dupuytren's contracture
_____ 6. Convex thoracic curve
_____ 7. Inversion of the foot 30°
_____ 8. Convex cervical curve
_____ 9. Ulnar deviation 55°
_____ 10. Hyperextension of the neck
_____ 11. Nontender masseter muscle
_____ 12. Shoulder internal rotation 90°
_____ 13. Warm hands for the nurse
_____ 14. Wrist extension 70°
_____ 15. Firm and stable hip joint
_____ 16. Hallux valgus
_____ 17. Muscle Strength 5
_____ 18. Genu varum
_____ 19. Elbow flexion 160°
_____ 20. Fluid collected in the suprapatellar bursa

FACTORS THAT INFLUENCE PHYSICAL ASSESSMENT FINDINGS

Fill in the blank(s) to complete each statement.

1. Arches in the feet develop during the _____ years.
2. Lordosis of the _____ progresses in the pregnant female to compensate for the growing fetus.
3. Osteoporosis develops more frequently in _____.
4. The nurse should consider _____ _____ if a client has a history of frequent fractures or musculoskeletal trauma.
5. Longitudinal bone growth ends at _____ years of age.
6. Asians and Caucasians have a higher incidence of _____.
7. The average person's height decreases by _____ to _____ inches from age 20 to 70.
8. Glucocorticoids may _____ bone density.
9. Estrogen and other hormones may _____ cartilage in the pregnant female.
10. The _____ _____ position stresses the hips, knees, and ankle joints of children.

Muscle Strength

Match the Muscle Strength rating in Column B with its characteristic in Column A. You may use each answer more than once.

Column A (Characteristics)

_____ 1. Full range of motion against gravity with moderate resistance
_____ 2. Trace
_____ 3. No muscle contraction
_____ 4. Full range of motion against gravity with full resistance
_____ 5. Fair
_____ 6. Full range of motion without gravity (passive) motion
_____ 7. Full range of motion with gravity
_____ 8. Palpable muscle contraction but no movement
_____ 9. Normal
_____ 10. Good

Column B (Rating)

A. Five
B. Four
C. Three
D. Two
E. One
F. Zero

Abnormal Findings

Write the name of each musculoskeletal disorder on the first line next to each illustration. On the second line, write one associated characteristic.

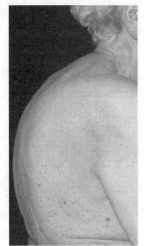

1. _____

   _____

Dr. P. Marazzi/Photo Researchers, Inc.

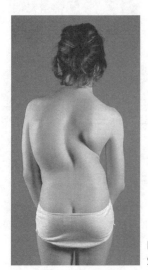

2. _____

   _____

Princess Margaret Rose Orthopaedic Hospital, Edinburgh,
Scotland/Science Photo Library/Photo Researchers, Inc.

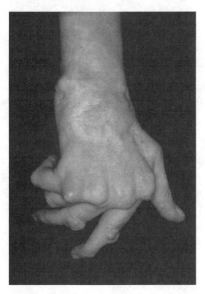

3. _____

   _____

Princess Margaret Rose Orthopaedic Hospital/Photo Researchers, Inc.

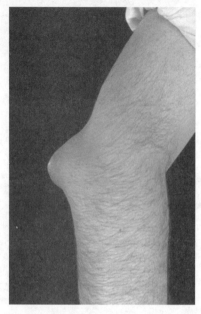

4. _____

_____

Medical-On-Line Ltd.

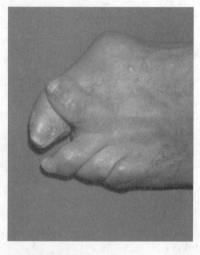

5. _____

_____

Dr. P. Marazzi/Photo Researchers, Inc.

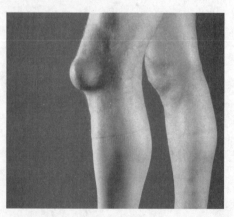

6. _____

_____

Princess Margaret Rose Orthopaedic Hospital/
Photo Researchers, Inc.

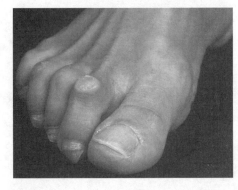

7. _____

_____

M. English/Stockphoto.com/Medichrome/
The Stock Shop, Inc.

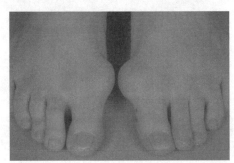

8. _____

_____

Biophoto Associates/Science Source/
Photo Researchers, Inc.

APPLICATION OF THE CRITICAL THINKING PROCESS

Part 1

Read the scenario below and then answer the questions that follow in the space provided.

Michelle is an 18-year-old girl who plays varsity basketball and volleyball at her high school. She has been playing sports since she was 5 years old. During a championship volleyball game, Michelle jumped up to block the ball and landed hard on her right knee. She states she felt her knee "pop" when she landed. She complained of extreme pain and difficulty with movement. She had to be removed from the game and brought to the school nurse because of edema at the injury site. Michelle begins to cry because it is too painful to move or bear weight on the right leg and states "My leg feels wobbly."

Michelle's past medical history is two sprained left ankles and a fractured right wrist. She has just completed her menstrual period 2 days ago. She takes a multivitamin daily.

Physical assessment reveals a well-developed female 5'9'', weighing 129 lb. The skin on her right knee is warm and dry. The color is consistent with the rest of her body. Her gait is unsteady, and she appears to hop on the left foot to avoid weight bearing on the right leg. She has limited ROM because of the pain. She states that when she is not moving her right knee, the pain is a 4 to 5 on a scale of 0 to 10, but when she moves it the pain increases to a 9 to 10.

The nurse suspects that Michelle has injured her right anterior cruciate ligament (RACL). The nurse calls for an ambulance to take her to the emergency department.

1. List three pieces of subjective data provided in this scenario.

   1. _____

   2. _____

   3. _____

2. List three pieces of objective data provided in this scenario.

1. _____

2. _____

3. _____

3. What further information should be collected in order to complete the pain assessment for this client?

4. List two reasons why it is important to assess this client's last menstrual period if her injury is musculoskeletal.

1. _____

2. _____

5. List two risk factors for an ACL injury for this client.

1. _____

2. _____

6. The client is told that she will need to ambulate with crutches until she has a surgical repair. The nurse will need to teach her how to use the crutches with no weight bearing on the right foot. Write a goal and three objectives that would be appropriate for this teaching plan.

Goal:

Objectives:

1. _____

2. _____

3. _____

Part 2

View the photograph below and answer the questions that follow.

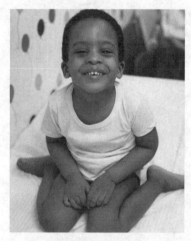

© Judy Braginsky

1. What is the name of this position? _____

2. The nurse notices a 2-year-old sitting in this position while playing a game.
What should the nurse tell the parents regarding this finding? Provide a rationale.

HEALTHY PEOPLE 2020

Read the *Healthy People 2020* objective and answer the questions that follow in the space provided.

A *Healthy People 2020* objective is:

Reduce the proportion of adults with osteoporosis.

1. List five focused questions that should be asked to determine a client's risk for osteoporosis.

   1. _____
   2. _____
   3. _____
   4. _____
   5. _____

2. A client with osteoporosis is at great risk for fractures. A fall assessment may be necessary to prevent such injury. Perform a search to find a fall assessment tool (you may use the Internet, health-related databases, etc.).

   1. State the name of the fall assessment tool: _____
   2. State the source: _____
   3. What are the elements that put a client at higher risk for falls, according to your tool? _____
   _____
   4. How can a home health nurse utilize this tool in order to prevent falls in the older adult population? _____
   _____
   5. How can a staff nurse in a postsurgical unit utilize this tool in order to prevent falls in a client who is recovering
   from surgery? _____
   _____

3. Discuss how an occupational nurse can use this objective to promote and maintain the health of the client.

ASSESSMENT AND DOCUMENTATION

Perform an assessment of the musculoskeletal system on your lab partner and document your findings on the following documentation form.

MUSCULOSKELETAL SYSTEM

Name:_____ Date:_____

Age: _____ Gender: _____

FOCUSED INTERVIEW

Reason for today's visit: _____

General Questions

Describe your mobility:

   Today: _____

   2 months ago: _____

   2 years ago: _____

Are you able to carry out all of your daily activities? _____

What is your current weight? _____

Allergies: _____

Recent illness: _____

Current medical conditions: _____

Past injuries: _____

Have you ever had a broken bone? _____

   How was it repaired? _____

Have you ever been in a motor vehicle accident? No _____ Yes _____ Explain _____

Have you ever experienced any type of serious injury? No _____ Yes _____ Explain _____

Have you ever experienced any penetrating wounds (nail, sharp object, gunshot, etc.)? _____

Have you noticed any changes in your gait in the past 6 months? _____

Have you experienced a fall in the past 6 months? _____

Do you walk with a cane, walker, or other assistive device? _____

Do you take any medications? _____

   Prescription: _____

   OTC: _____

Do you take calcium supplements, glucosamine, or any other type of over-the-counter supplements for your musculoskeletal system? _____

Have you ever had a bone density scan? _____

   What were the results? _____

Describe any disorders you have related to your musculoskeletal system: _____

_____

Describe any disorders your family members may have related to the musculoskeletal system: _____

_____

What kind of work do you or did you do? _____

Describe any heavy lifting you do more than once per week:

   10–25 lb: _____

   26–50 lb: _____

   Greater than 50 lb: _____

Do you wear any supportive devices when you lift heavy objects? _____

Have you ever received formal training on the proper techniques for heavy lifting? _____

_____

Describe your hobbies and/or athletic activities: _____

Do you exercise? _____

   Frequency: _____

   Type: _____

Age-Related Questions

Infants and Children

Were you told about any trauma to the infant during labor and delivery? _____

Did the baby require resuscitation at delivery? _____

Have you noticed any deformity of the child's spine or limbs, or feet and toes? _____

Describe any dislocation or broken bones and treatment. _____

School-Age Children

Does the child play any sports at school or after school? _____

Pregnant Females

Describe any back pain you are experiencing: _____

Older Adults

Have you noticed muscle weakness over the past few months? _____

Have you fallen in the past 6 months? _____

Do you use any walking aids? _____

For postmenopausal females: Do you take calcium supplements? _____

Symptoms or Behaviors

Do you now or have you ever had:

   Joints:

      Swelling: _____

      Heat: _____

      Redness: _____

      ROM: _____

      Stiffness: _____

      Pain: _____

   Muscles:

      Swelling: _____

      Heat: _____

      Redness: _____

      Weakness: _____

      Pain: _____

PHYSICAL ASSESSMENT

Vital signs: _____ BP _____ HR _____ RR _____ Temp

GENERAL SURVEY

Overall appearance: _____

Posture: _____

Position: _____

Gait: _____

Deformities: _____

TEMPOROMANDIBULAR JOINT

Inspection

Symmetry: Right: _____   Left: _____

Deformities: Right: _____   Left: _____

Swelling: Right: _____   Left: _____

Palpation

Tenderness: Right: _____   Left: _____

Muscles: Right: _____   Left: _____

Strength: Right: _____   Left: _____

Pain: Right: _____   Left: _____

ROM

Opening and closing jaw: _____

Protraction and retraction: _____

Side-to-side movement: _____

Other: _____

SHOULDERS

Inspection

Symmetry: Right: _____   Left: _____

Deformities: Right: _____   Left: _____

Swelling: Right: _____   Left: _____

Palpation

Tenderness: Right: _____   Left: _____

Muscles: Right: _____   Left: _____

Strength: Right: _____   Left: _____

Pain: Right: _____   Left: _____

ROM

Abduction: Right: _____   Left: _____

Adduction: Right: _____   Left: _____

Horizontal forward flexion: Right: _____   Left: _____

Horizontal backward flexion: Right: _____   Left: _____

Circumduction: Right: _____   Left: _____

External rotation: Right: _____   Left: _____

Internal rotation: Right: _____   Left: _____

ELBOWS

Inspection

Symmetry: Right: _____   Left: _____

Deformities: Right: _____   Left: _____

Swelling: Right: _____   Left: _____

Palpation

Tenderness: Right: _____   Left: _____

Muscles: Right: _____   Left: _____

Strength: Right: _____   Left: _____

Pain: Right: _____   Left: _____

ROM

Flexion of the forearm: Right: _____   Left: _____

Extension of the forearm: Right: _____   Left: _____

Supination of the forearm
and hand: Right: _____   Left: _____

Pronation of the forearm
and hand: Right: _____   Left: _____

WRISTS AND HANDS

Inspection

Symmetry: Right: _____   Left: _____

Deformities: Right: _____   Left: _____

Swelling: Right: _____   Left: _____

Palpation

Tenderness: Right: _____   Left: _____

Muscles: Right: _____   Left: _____

Strength: Right: _____   Left: _____

Pain: Right: _____   Left: _____

ROM
Wrist

Flexion: Right: _____   Left: _____

Extension: Right: _____   Left: _____

Hyperextension: Right: _____   Left: _____

Radial deviation: Right: _____   Left: _____

Ulnar deviation: Right: _____   Left: _____

Fingers

Abduction: Right: _____   Left: _____

Extension: Right: _____   Left: _____

Hyperextension: Right: _____   Left: _____

Flexion: Right: _____   Left: _____

Circumduction: Right: _____   Left: _____

Thumb

Extension: Right: _____   Left: _____

Flexion: Right: _____   Left: _____

Opposition: Right: _____   Left: _____

Phalen's test: _____

Tinel's sign: _____

Other: _____

HIP
Inspection

Symmetry: Right: _____   Left: _____

Deformities: Right: _____   Left: _____

Swelling: Right: _____   Left: _____

Palpation

Tenderness: Right: _____   Left: _____

Muscles: Right: _____   Left: _____

Strength: Right: _____   Left: _____

Pain: Right: _____   Left: _____

ROM

Extension: Right: _____   Left: _____

Hyperextension: Right: _____   Left: _____

Flexion with knee flexed: Right: _____   Left: _____

Flexion with knee extended: Right: _____   Left: _____

Internal rotation: Right: _____   Left: _____

External rotation: Right: _____   Left: _____
Abduction: Right: _____   Left: _____
Adduction: Right: _____   Left: _____

KNEE

Inspection

Symmetry: Right: _____   Left: _____
Deformities: Right: _____   Left: _____
Swelling: Right: _____   Left: _____

Palpation

Tenderness: Right: _____   Left: _____
Muscles: Right: _____   Left: _____
Strength: Right: _____   Left: _____
Pain: Right: _____   Left: _____
Bulge sign: Right: _____   Left: _____
Ballottement: Right: _____   Left: _____

ROM

Flexion: Right: _____   Left: _____
Extension: Right: _____   Left: _____
Hyperextension: Right: _____   Left: _____

ANKLES AND FEET

Inspection

Symmetry: Right: _____   Left: _____
Deformities: Right: _____   Left: _____
Swelling: Right: _____   Left: _____

Palpation

Tenderness: Right: _____   Left: _____
Muscles: Right: _____   Left: _____
Achilles tendon: Right: _____   Left: _____
Strength: Right: _____   Left: _____
Pain: Right: _____   Left: _____

ROM

Ankle

Dorsiflexion: Right: _____   Left: _____
Plantar flexion: Right: _____   Left: _____
Inversion of foot: Right: _____   Left: _____
Eversion of foot: Right: _____   Left: _____

Toes

Extension: Right: _____   Left: _____

Flexion: Right: _____   Left: _____

Abduction: Right: _____   Left: _____

Adduction: Right: _____   Left: _____

SPINE

Inspection

Symmetry: _____

Deformities: _____

Swelling: _____

Curvature: _____

Palpation

Tenderness: _____

Muscles: _____

Achilles tendon: _____

Strength: _____

Pain: _____

ROM

Neck (Cervical spine)

Flexion: _____

Extension: _____

Hyperextension: _____

Lateral flexion: _____

Rotation: _____

Spine

Lateral flexion: _____

Extension: _____

Flexion: _____

Rotation: _____

Other: _____

NCLEX®-STYLE REVIEW QUESTIONS

Read each question carefully. Choose the best answer for each question.

1. The head of the femur placed into the acetabulum forms the:
   1. hip joint
   2. shoulder
   3. elbow
   4. knee

2. A middle-age client seeks clarification from the nurse about the difference between a muscle strain and a muscle sprain. The nurse explains that: (Select all that apply.)
    1. a strain includes the partial tear or overstretching of a muscle or tendon
    2. a sprain includes a tear or overstretching of a ligament
    3. a strain is medical terminology for a fatigued muscle
    4. a sprain is medical terminology for a ruptured tendon
    5. a strain is a term for inflammation and weakness in skeletal muscles

3. The nurse should ask the client to only flex and extend the knees because they have what type of joints?
    1. Hinge
    2. Saddle
    3. Pivot
    4. Condyloid

4. Inversion and eversion refer to movements of what body part?
    1. Hand
    2. Arm
    3. Thumb
    4. Foot

5. While assessing the back of a newborn, the nurse sees a tuft of hair at the base of the spine. The nurse suspects which condition?
    1. Allis sign
    2. Genu valgum
    3. Spina bifida
    4. Genu varum

6. A 62-year-old male reports to the clinic complaining of a flare-up of his gout. Which signs and symptoms does the nurse anticipate finding during an assessment? (Select all that apply.)
    1. Swelling in the affected joint
    2. Inflammation in the affected joint
    3. A yellow discoloration to the skin
    4. A gritty texture to the skin
    5. Pain in the affected joint

7. When performing a musculoskeletal assessment, the nurse must remember to:
    1. use as many client position changes as possible
    2. work distal to proximal
    3. attempt to move a joint about 5 degrees farther when pain is elicited
    4. demonstrate the movements

8. When rating muscle strength as a 4 on a scale from 0 to 5, what is the nurse's best description of the findings for the client?
    1. Poor
    2. Fair
    3. Good
    4. Excellent

9. The nurse performs Phalen's test on a client with carpal tunnel syndrome. The nurse expects pain to radiate to which area?
    1. Legs
    2. Knees
    3. Shoulder
    4. Spine

10. A nurse who suspects a client may have carpal tunnel syndrome may decide to use which of the following assessment techniques? (Select all that apply.)
    1. Phalen's test
    2. Bulge test
    3. Tinel's sign
    4. Ballottement test
    5. Straight leg raise test

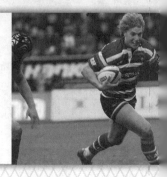

The mind, once expanded to the dimensions of larger ideas, never returns to its original size.
—Oliver Wendell Holmes

The neurologic system includes reflexes, movements, sensations, and the senses. The nurse must have knowledge of the ways in which the neurologic system affects human function in order to determine if an assessment indicates abnormalities within this system. This chapter will focus on gathering both subjective and objective data related to the neurologic system, as well as analysis of the data collected.

OBJECTIVES

At the completion of these exercises, you will be able to:

1. Review the anatomy and physiology of the neurologic system.
2. Identify the correct techniques for assessment of the neurologic system.
3. Analyze subjective and objective data related to assessment of the neurologic system.
4. Recognize factors that can influence assessment findings.
5. Apply critical thinking in analysis of a case study.
6. Relate *Healthy People 2020* objectives to the neurologic system.
7. Assess the neurologic system on a laboratory partner.
8. Document an assessment of the neurologic system.
9. Complete NCLEX®-style review questions related to the assessment of the neurologic system.

ANATOMY & PHYSIOLOGY REVIEW

1. For each of the following diagrams, label the structures as indicated by each line.

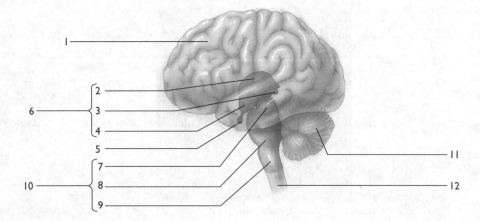

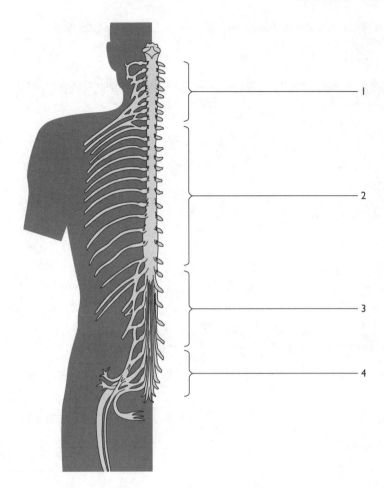

2. Match each lobe of the cerebrum in Column B to its function in Column A. Some lobes will be used more than once.

Column A

_____ 1. Creation of abstract ideas

_____ 2. Interpretation of visual stimuli

_____ 3. Awareness of sensation

_____ 4. Concern for others

_____ 5. Contains the olfactory cortex

_____ 6. Awareness of somatosensory stimuli

_____ 7. Controls intellect

_____ 8. Interpretation of auditory stimuli

_____ 9. Controls speech

_____ 10. Controls reasoning

Column B

A. Frontal lobe
B. Parietal lobe
C. Temporal lobe
D. Occipital lobe

3. Read the scenario below and then answer the questions that follow in the space provided.

A 3-year-old boy touches the hot oven while his mother is baking cupcakes. He quickly pulls his hand away and begins to cry. The mother jumps up from her seat and runs to her son in a panic.

1. List the components of the reflex arc that occurred when the boy touched the stove.

2. What portion of the brain is responsible for the boy's emotional response of crying?

3. List four physiologic changes that may be noted during the fight-or-flight response of the mother.

   1.

   2.

   3.

   4.

4. Identify the cranial nerve(s) responsible for each activity by placing the name and corresponding number next to the activities below. More than one nerve may be responsible for an activity.

   1. Sticking out the tongue

      Name _____

      Number _____

   2. Swallowing lunch

      Name _____

      Number _____

   3. Seeing a rainbow

      Name _____

      Number _____

   4. Rolling the eyes

      Name _____

      Number _____

   5. Singing a song

      Name _____

      Number _____

   6. Feeling a sharp object on the right cheek

      Name _____

      Number _____

   7. Listening to music

      Name _____

      Number _____

   8. Raising the eyebrows

      Name _____

      Number _____

   9. Smelling a flower

      Name _____

      Number _____

   10. Shrugging the shoulders

      Name _____

      Number _____

   11. Constricting the pupils

      Name _____

      Number _____

   12. Walking on a balance beam

      Name _____

      Number _____

   13. Clenching the teeth

      Name _____

      Number _____

   14. Tasting a strawberry

      Name _____

      Number _____

   15. Smiling at a friend

      Name _____

      Number _____

   16. Gagging

      Name _____

      Number _____

ASSESSMENT TECHNIQUES

Review each assessment technique. If the technique is correct, circle the number. If the technique is incorrect, write the correct assessment technique on the line provided.

1. To assess the client's sensorium, the nurse should ask the client to determine the date, time, place, and reason for today's visit.

   _____

   _____

2. The client should close both eyes and one nare when having cranial nerve II (two) assessed.

   _____

   _____

3. When testing motor function of cranial nerve V (five), the client should be asked to tightly clench the teeth.

   _____

   _____

4. Convergence and accommodation should be assessed for sensory function of cranial nerve V.

   _____

   _____

5. When assessing the client's gait, the nurse must be sure the client is looking straight ahead and not at the floor.

   _____

   _____

6. The nurse should stand in front of the client when performing the Romberg test.

   _____

   _____

7. A rapid alternating action can be assessed by asking the client to touch the thumb to each finger in sequence with increasing pace.

   _____

   _____

8. When testing for graphesthesia the client should keep both eyes open.

   _____

   _____

9. When assessing the brachioradialis reflex, the nurse should briskly strike the tendon toward the radius about 1 inch above the wrist.

   _____

   _____

10. The flat end of the reflex hammer is used to assess the Babinski reflex.

   _____

   _____

ASSESSMENT FINDINGS

Read each assessment finding. Identify the finding as normal or abnormal by writing an "N" for normal or an "A" for abnormal on each line provided.

_____ 1. Asymmetrical facial movements

_____ 2. Hoarseness of voice

_____ 3. Glasgow Coma Scale 3

_____ 4. Dysphagia

_____ 5. 14 triceps reflex

_____ 6. Short-term memory intact

_____ 7. Nuchal rigidity

_____ 8. Ataxic gait

_____ 9. Dystonia

_____ 10. Two-point discrimination at 10 cm in the lower leg

_____ 11. Vertigo

_____ 12. Articulate speech

_____ 13. Anosmia

_____ 14. Negative Romberg

_____ 15. Stepping reflex age 5 months

_____ 16. Auditory hallucinations

_____ 17. Glasgow Coma Scale 14

_____ 18. 12 brachioradialis reflex

_____ 19. Anesthesia

_____ 20. Monotone voice

FACTORS THAT INFLUENCE PHYSICAL ASSESSMENT FINDINGS

Fill in the blank(s) to complete each statement.

1. Hyperactive reflexes may indicate _____ _____ _____ in the pregnant female.

2. African Americans have a higher incidence of hypertension, thus increasing their risk for _____.

3. During pregnancy, as the uterus enlarges, it may exert pressure on the pelvic nerves, causing pain, numbness, or tingling to travel to the _____.

4. Cerebral disease should be considered if a newborn has a/an _____ cry.

5. The growth of the nervous system is very _____ during the fetal period.

6. The Moro and sucking reflexes are considered _____ reflexes in the newborn.

7. Peripheral neuropathy and encephalopathy may be caused by _____ poisoning.

8. In the United States, _____ _____ have higher rates of Alzheimer's disease than Caucasians.

9. The senses tend to _____ in the older adult.

10. Research suggests that toxins such as carbon monoxide may cause some cases of _____ _____.

APPLICATION OF THE CRITICAL THINKING PROCESS

Read each of the scenarios below and then answer the questions that follow in the space provided.

SCENARIO 1

Melanie is a 32-year-old female who is in the intensive care unit after a drug overdose with suicidal intent. When the nurse enters the room to assess her, the nurse notes that Melanie's eyes are closed. When the nurse calls her name, Melanie opens her lids but does not focus on any specific object. The nurse informs Melanie that her intravenous site is due to be changed and asks Melanie if she can move her left arm closer to the edge of the bed; Melanie does not respond. When the nurse attempts to insert the angiocatheter into the basilic vein, Melanie pulls back her arm and groans. The nurse asks Melanie if she is feeling pain. Melanie again just moans and closes her eyes.

1. List the three areas of the Glasgow Coma Scale.

    1.

    2.

    3.

2. Use the Glasgow Coma Scale to assess Melanie's level of consciousness.

3. What are the implications of your findings?

SCENARIO 2

Mrs. Sharon Sanchez, a 42-year-old Hispanic female, has been married for 15 years and has a 10-year-old son. She suffered a head injury 20 years ago in a motor vehicle crash as an unbelted passenger. She was treated and released after 2 days of observation for a concussion. At this time she works as a hairstylist in a local beauty salon. She takes no medications except for an occasional Excedrin for the migraine headaches she has been having for the past 3 weeks. She denies the use of alcohol and tobacco.

Mrs. Sanchez's chief complaint is a sharp pain above and behind her right eye. Her husband states "her face just doesn't look right to me." Upon physical assessment, the nurse notes ptosis of the right eyelid and mild unilateral right facial weakness. Her speech is articulate and the motor movements of her upper extremities are symmetrical and strong.

1. Use OLDCART & ICE to identify five focused interview questions that the nurse should ask this client.

    1.

    2.

    3.

    4.

    5.

2. Perform a web search through the National Institutes of Health (NIH) for the NIH stroke scale. List the performance indicators for this scale.

3. Perform a web search for the Cincinnati Stroke Scale. List the performance indicators for this scale.

4. Evaluate the two scales in relationship to ease of use and the healthcare setting.

5. After careful assessment and diagnostic testing, an unruptured brain aneurysm has been detected. Name at least three other signs or symptoms that may be noted for this diagnosis. (Additional resources may be necessary.)

   1.

   2.

   3.

6. Identify and prioritize two nursing diagnoses for this client.

   1.

   2.

HEALTHY PEOPLE 2020

Read the *Healthy People 2020* objective and answer the questions that follow in the space provided. (Additional resources may be necessary.)

A *Healthy People 2020* objective is:

Reduce traumatic brain injury morbidity and mortality.

1. A concussion is considered a mild traumatic brain injury. List five signs and symptoms of a concussion.

   1. _____
   2. _____
   3. _____
   4. _____
   5. _____

2. According to the Centers for Disease Control and Prevention, children between the ages of 0 and 19 years of age are at highest risk for traumatic brain injury. List three reasons that support this risk.

   1. _____
   2. _____
   3. _____

3. Discuss how a nurse can use this objective to promote and maintain the health of the client.

ASSESSMENT AND DOCUMENTATION

Perform an assessment of the neurologic system on your lab partner and document your findings on the following documentation form.

NEUROLOGIC SYSTEM

Name:_____Date:_____

Age: _____ Gender: _____

FOCUSED INTERVIEW

Reason for today's visit: _____

_____

General Questions

Describe any difficulties you have carrying out your activities of daily living: _____

_____

Do you have any chronic diseases such as diabetes or hypertension? _____

Do any members of your family now have, or have they ever had, a neurologic problem or disease?

_____

Have you ever been diagnosed with a neurologic illness? No _____ Yes _____ Explain _____

_____

Have you ever had an injury to your head, neck, or back? No _____ Yes _____ Explain _____

_____

Allergies: _____

Recent illness: _____

Current medical conditions: _____

Medications (prescription and over the counter, including any herbal or vitamin supplements):

_____

Past injuries: _____

Have you noticed any changes in your gait in the past

    6 days? _____

    6 weeks? _____

    6 months? _____

Do you walk with a cane, walker, or other assistive device? _____

Have you experienced a fall in the past 6 months? _____

Do you drop things easily? _____

Do you consider yourself clumsy? _____

Do you wear a helmet when biking, skateboarding, skiing? _____

Do you wear a seat belt in a car? _____

Do you now or have you ever used recreational drugs or alcohol? _____

Do you live in a home built before 1978? _____

Are you exposed to any toxic chemicals at home or at work? No _____ Yes _____ Explain _____

_____

Have you ever found a tick on your body or pet? _____

Age-Related Questions

Infants and Children

List any health problems and medications, alcohol, or drugs used during pregnancy: _____

Ever had a seizure? _____

Noticed any clumsiness? _____

Lead-based paint in the home? _____

How is the child doing in school? _____

Pregnant Females

History of seizures? _____

Taking vitamins or nutritional supplements? _____

Older Adults

Does it take more time to perform tasks than 2 years ago? _____ 5 yrs ago? _____ Explain.

Do you have trouble walking when you stand up? _____

Notice any tremors? _____

List safety features in the home: _____

Symptoms or Behaviors

Do you now or have you ever had:

Fainting: _____

Dizziness: _____

Light-headedness: _____

Seizures: _____

Tremors: _____

Visual disturbances: _____

Hearing difficulties: _____

Changes in your sense of taste: _____

Changes in your sense of smell: _____

Numbness or tingling sensations: _____

Headaches: _____

Pain: _____

Memory difficulties: _____

Speech difficulties: _____

PHYSICAL ASSESSMENT

Vital signs: _____ BP _____ HR _____ RR _____ Temp

MENTAL STATUS

Overall appearance: _____

Hygiene: _____

Grooming: _____

Posture: _____

Body language: _____

Facial expressions: _____

Speech:

    Articulation: _____

    Tone: _____

    Volume: _____

Ability to follow directions: _____

Orientation:

    Date: _____

    Time: _____

    Place: _____

    Reason for being evaluated: _____

Memory:

    Short term: _____

    Long term: _____

    Ability to calculate: _____

    Abstract thinking: _____

    Mood and emotional state: _____

    Perceptions and thought processes: _____

    Judgment: _____

Cranial Nerves

CN	Assessment	Normal	Abnormal	Comments
I	Smell and odor distinction			
II	Distant vision			
	Near vision			
III, IV, VI	PERRLA			
	EOM			
V	Sensations			
	Corneal reflex			
	Motor function			
VII	Facial movements symmetrical			
	Muscle strength of upper face			

CN	Assessment	Normal	Abnormal	Comments
	Muscle strength of lower face			
	Taste			
	Corneal reflex			
VIII	Weber			
	Rinne			
	Whisper			
	Romberg			
IX, X	Swallowing			
	Gag reflex			
	Taste			
	Voice			
XI	Turn head			
	Turn head against resistance			
	Shrug shoulders			
	Shrug shoulders against resistance			
XII	Tongue movement			
	Tongue movement against resistance			

MOTOR FUNCTION

Gait: _____

    Heel to toe: _____

    Tiptoe: _____

    Heel: _____

Romberg test: _____

Finger-to-nose:

    Right: _____   Left: _____

Rapid alternating movements:

    Right: _____   Left: _____

Heel-to-shin:

    Right: _____   Left: _____

SENSORY FUNCTION

Light touch:

    Location: _____

    Finding: _____

Sharp and dull:

    Location: _____

    Finding: _____

Temperature:

    Location: _____

    Finding: _____

Vibration:

    Location: _____

    Finding: _____

Stereognosis:

    Location: _____

    Finding: _____

Graphesthesia:

    Location: _____

    Finding: _____

Two-point discrimination: _____

    Lower leg: _____

    Upper leg: _____

    Wrist area: _____

    Upper part of arm: _____

Topognosis: _____

    Location: _____

    Finding: _____

REFLEXES

Biceps

    R   0   1+   2+   3+   4+

    Comments: _____

    L   0   1+   2+   3+   4+

    Comments: _____

Triceps

    R   0   1+   2+   3+   4+

    Comments: _____

    L   0   1+   2+   3+   4+

    Comments: _____

Brachioradialis

    R   0   1+   2+   3+   4+

    Comments: _____

    L   0   1+   2+   3+   4+

    Comments: _____

Patellar

    R   0   1+   2+   3+   4+

    Comments: _____

    L   0   1+   2+   3+   4+

    Comments: _____

Achilles

    R   0   1+   2+   3+   4+

    Comments: _____

    L   0   1+   2+   3+   4+

    Comments: _____

Plantar

    R   0   1+   2+   3+   4+

    Comments: _____

    L   0   1+   2+   3+   4+

    Comments: _____

Abdominal:

    RLQ: _____

    RUQ: _____

    LUQ: _____

    LLQ: _____

Glasgow Coma Scale

GLASGOW COMA SCALE
BEST EYE-OPENING RESPONSE 4 = Spontaneously 3 = To speech 2 = To pain 1 = No response **(Record "C" if eyes closed by swelling.)**
BEST MOTOR RESPONSE to painful stimuli 6 = Obeys verbal command 5 = Localizes pain 4 = Flexion—withdrawal 3 = Flexion—abnormal 2 = Extension—abnormal 1 = No response **(Record best upper limb response.)**
BEST VERBAL RESPONSE 5 = Oriented ×3 4 = Conversation—confused 3 = Speech—inappropriate 2 = Sounds—incomprehensible 1 = No response **(Record "E" if endotracheal tube in place, "T" if tracheostomy tube in place.)**

Best eye-opening response: _____ Best motor response: _____ Best verbal response: _____

NCLEX®-STYLE REVIEW QUESTIONS

Read each question carefully. Choose the best answer for each question.

1. The nurse identifies which portion of the brain as the one responsible for all conscious behavior?
    1. Cerebellum
    2. Brain stem
    3. Cerebrum
    4. Central nervous system

2. The nurse understands that a positive Babinski reflex is a normal finding in:
    1. all clients
    2. an infant
    3. an adult client
    4. a pregnant client

3. The nurse notes which of the following neurologic findings as part of the normal aging process in the older adult client? (Select all that apply.)
    1. Increased deep tendon reflexes
    2. Decreased visual acuity
    3. Decreased reaction time
    4. Erect posture
    5. Tremor

4. The nurse will use which of the following questions during the focused neurologic interview of the client? (Select all that apply.)
    1. "Have you ever experienced a seizure?"
    2. "Do you have numbness or tingling in your arms or legs?"
    3. "Have you ever had an injury to your head?"
    4. "Have you experienced any redness or swelling to your eyes?"
    5. "Do you consume alcohol?"

5. Which of the following is/are true about the physical assessment of the neurologic system? (Select all that apply.)
    1. The nurse should proceed cephalocaudal and proximal to distal
    2. It begins after the focused interview
    3. Several assessments may occur at one time
    4. It will always require three sessions with an elderly client
    5. The nurse will use inspection, palpation, auscultation, and percussion in the neurologic assessment of a client

6. When assessing the Achilles tendon reflex, the expected response would be:
    1. plantar flexion of the foot
    2. dorsiflexion of the foot
    3. fanning of the toes, with dorsiflexion of the great toe
    4. no response

7. The components of the Glasgow Coma Scale are: (Select all that apply.)
    1. eye response
    2. sensory response
    3. motor response
    4. verbal response
    5. reflexes

8. When assessing for cortical disease in a client, the nurse should perform which of the following tests?
    1. Deep tendon reflex testing
    2. Stereognosis
    3. Rapid alternating actions of the upper extremity
    4. Romberg's test

9. An older adult female client is brought to the medical clinic by her daughter. The client's daughter states, "I think my mother is showing signs of Alzheimer's disease." Based on the daughter's statement, the nurse would expect that the client is showing which group of signs and symptoms?

    1. A flat affect, diplopia, and memory loss

    2. Memory loss, confusion, and periods of disorientation

    3. Disorientation, shuffled gait, and dystonia

    4. Tics and tremors, confusion, and diplopia

10. When assessing the deep tendon reflexes on a client, the nurse notes they are brisk. The nurse documents this finding as:

    1. 1+

    2. 2+

    3. 3+

    4. 4+

27 ⟩ The Pregnant Female

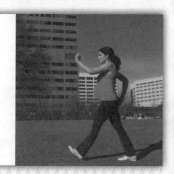

A mother is she who can take the place of all others but whose place no one else can take.
—Cardinal Mermillod

This chapter is designed to help you develop the skills needed for the assessment of the pregnant female.

The data collected provide a basis for the planning of nursing care.

OBJECTIVES

At the completion of these exercises, you will be able to:

1. Describe anatomic and physiologic variations in the pregnant client.
2. Write focused interview questions related to pregnancy.
3. Using Nägele's rule and last menstrual period, calculate estimated date of delivery.
4. Describe uterine size and fetal position of the pregnant female.
5. Explain abnormal findings associated with pregnancy.
6. Identify risk factors concerning pregnancy for women of various age groups.
7. Apply critical thinking in analysis of a case study.
8. Respond to NCLEX®-style questions related to assessment of pregnant and postpartum females.

ANATOMIC AND PHYSIOLOGIC CHANGES OF PREGNANCY

List anatomic and physiologic changes seen in a pregnant female for the following categories.

1. Weight: _____
   _____
   _____

2. Skin, hair, and nails: _____
   _____
   _____

3. Cardiovascular system: _____
   _____
   _____

4. Respiratory system: _____
   _____
   _____

5. Gastrointestinal system: _____
   _____
   _____

6. Urinary system: _____

_____

_____

7. Reproductive system: _____

_____

_____

FOCUSED INTERVIEW

1. Write five focused interview questions related to assessing a pregnant female at the first visit to the obstetric office.

   1. _____

   2. _____

   3. _____

   4. _____

   5. _____

2. Write five focused interview questions to ask at the next or follow-up visit.

   1. _____

   2. _____

   3. _____

   4. _____

   5. _____

ASSESSMENT OF FETAL GROWTH

1. Calculate the estimated date of delivery using Nägele's rule for the following LMPs.

   1. July 20: _____

   2. January 3: _____

   3. November 12: _____

2. Describe the height of the uterus for the following number of weeks of gestation.

   1. 20 weeks of gestation: _____

   2. 28 weeks of gestation: _____

   3. 36 weeks of gestation: _____

FETAL LIE, PRESENTATION, AND POSITION

Answer the following questions that support the fetus in the uterus.

1. Define Leopold's maneuvers. _____

_____

_____

2. Match the data in Column A with the Leopold's maneuvers found in Column B.

<u>**Column A**</u>   <u>**Column B**</u>

_____ **1.** A longitudinal lie will find the head of the fetus in the fundus   **A.** First
of the uterus   **B.** Second

_____ **2.** Identifies the depth of the presenting part in the pelvis   **C.** Third

_____ **3.** Location of the fetal back   **D.** Fourth

_____ **4.** Nothing in the fundus of the uterus indicates transverse lie

_____ **5.** Soft irregular mass in fetal breech

_____ **6.** A hard, round, independently movable mass is palpated in the
pelvis

_____ **7.** Fetal back against mother's back is a posterior position

_____ **8.** Identification of the presenting part of the uterus

_____ **9.** During palpation of the mother's abdomen, the fingers of the
nurse come together above the superior edge of the symphysis
pubis; the presenting part is floating

_____ **10.** Identification of fetal small parts on the left side of the mother

3. Identify fetal position in the following diagrams by using the accepted abbreviations.

1.

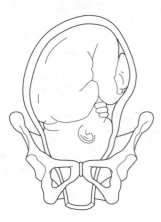

Answer _____

3.

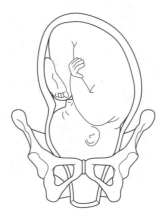

Answer _____

2.

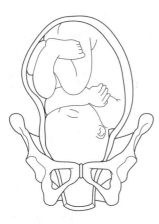

Answer _____

4.

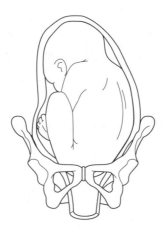

Answer _____

5.

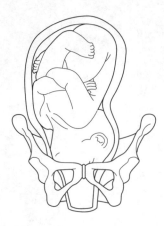

Answer _____

Source: Courtesy of Abbott Nutrition, Columbus, OH.

RISK FACTORS AND ABNORMAL FINDINGS

1. Describe five risk factors associated with pregnancy.

   1. _____
   2. _____
   3. _____
   4. _____
   5. _____

2. List or describe signs and symptoms of the following abnormal findings associated with pregnancy.

   1. Preeclampsia: _____
   _____
   _____

   2. Gestational diabetes: _____
   _____
   _____

   3. Preterm labor: _____
   _____
   _____

   4. Mood disorders: _____
   _____
   _____

APPLICATION OF THE CRITICAL THINKING PROCESS

Read each of the scenarios below and then answer the questions that follow in the space provided.

SCENARIO 1

A nurse in an obstetric clinic is caring for Ms. K. B., a 36-year-old with an obstetric history of spontaneous abortions at ages 30 and 32 and a preterm vaginal delivery at 35 weeks 2 years ago, who is pregnant again. Ms. K. B. states that her LMP was 2 months ago on 12/21. Ms. K. B. is a single mom to a toddler and works full time. Ms. K. B. reports to the nurse that her BP was elevated and she had swelling of the face, arms, and legs during the pregnancy 2 years ago.

1. Document Ms. K. B's gravidity and parity in obstetric terms.

2. Using Nägele's rule, calculate the expected date of confinement (EDC).

3. Identify four risk factors associated with Ms. K. B's pregnancy.

    1.

    2.

    3.

    4.

4. Identify three educational topics Ms. K. B. can benefit from.

    1.

    2.

    3.

5. State five objectives presented in *Healthy People 2020* that would apply to this client.

    1.

    2.

3.

4.

5.

6. Explain the following signs of pregnancy.

   1. Presumptive: _____

   2. Probable: _____

   3. Positive: _____

SCENARIO 2

The nurse is caring for D. K., a 23-year-old on the second postpartum day after a normal vaginal delivery and giving birth to a healthy newborn. D. K. had a second-degree vaginal tear during childbirth. D. K.'s obstetric history is gravida 1 and para 1. D. K. states that she is a single mother and that her mother agreed to help with the baby for a few weeks.

1. During assessment on the second postpartum day, the nurse observes that the fundal height is above the umbilicus and displaced to the right side of the abdomen. The nurse concludes that this may be the result of what?

   _____

2. What should be the nurse's next assessment, based on the above conclusion?

3. Based on D. K.'s obstetric history, identify three teaching–learning needs for this client.

   1.

   2.

   3.

4. When caring for this client, the nurse understands that the two most important causes of postpartum infection are

   _____ and _____.

NCLEX®-STYLE REVIEW QUESTIONS

Read each question carefully. Choose the best answer for each question.

1. For a woman with a 28-day menstrual cycle, ovulation begins on what day of the menstrual cycle?
   1. 1st day of the menstrual cycle
   2. 7th day of the menstrual cycle
   3. 14th day of the menstrual cycle
   4. 28th day of the menstrual cycle

2. An emergency department nurse is talking to a young female who states that she was sexually assaulted by a friend during a party the day before. The woman stated that "I felt so ashamed and dirty that I ran home and took a shower." What is the initial response of the nurse in this situation?
   1. "You may have destroyed the evidence by taking a shower."
   2. "Do you remember exactly what happened? Were you drunk?"
   3. "I understand that it was important for you to take a shower after what happened."
   4. "Do you have the clothes you were wearing at the time and have you washed them?"

3. The nurse assessing an antenatal client determines that the presumptive signs of pregnancy include which of the following? (Select all that apply.)
   1. Breast tenderness
   2. Amenorrhea
   3. Uterine enlargement
   4. Increased urinary frequency
   5. Quickening

4. Which of the following would be included when performing a postpartum assessment on a client who is first-day postpartum after a vaginal delivery? (Select all that apply.)
   1. Assess the breasts
   2. Assess the perineum
   3. Assess extremities
   4. Check vaginal discharge
   5. Assess fundal height

5. During the postpartum period, levels of which of the following hormones will sharply increase in a client and will aid in breast milk production?
   1. Prolactin
   2. Estrogen
   3. Human chorionic gonadotropin
   4. Human placental lactogen

6. A Muslim client who has just delivered states that she is hungry and requests food. The nurse should ensure that which of the following products are avoided in the meal?
   1. Beef
   2. Pork
   3. Milk
   4. Poultry

7. Place the different stages of fetal development in chronological order
   1. Vernix caseosa is seen
   2. Blastocyst development is complete
   3. Testes have descended into the scrotal sac
   4. Chambers of the heart have developed

8. A client shows up in the clinic and raises the concern that she might be pregnant. Elevation of the levels of which hormone will confirm her suspicion?
   1. Human chorionic gonadotropin
   2. Pitocin
   3. Estrogen
   4. Luteinizing hormone

9. Cardiac output in a pregnant female changes in what way?
   1. Increases along with stroke volume
   2. Decreases significantly
   3. Remains the same
   4. Increases, with no change in stroke volume

10. A woman who is 18 weeks pregnant and is complaining of lower abdominal pain may be experiencing which of the following conditions?
    1. Appendicitis
    2. Urinary tract infection
    3. Constipation
    4. Stretching of round ligament

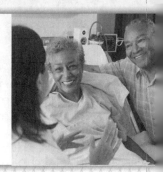

Accomplishment is easiest when we work the hardest, and it is hardest when we work the least.
—Author Unknown

This chapter is developed to help the student apply the principles of assessment to an individual in a state of health reflecting illness in a hospital setting. These principles could be applied across the age span and in any area of care.

OBJECTIVES

At the completion of these exercises, you will be able to:

1. Apply the nursing process to a client situation.
2. Utilize two assessment types the nurse will use when assessing a hospitalized client.
3. Identify expected findings from physical assessment of the respiratory status of clients across the age span.
4. Apply critical thinking in analysis of a case study.
5. Incorporate National Patient Safety Goals into hospitalized client care.
6. Document findings of a hospitalized client's rapid and routine (or initial) assessment.
7. Respond to NCLEX®-style questions related to assessment of a hospitalized client.

NURSING PROCESS

Read the scenario below and then answer the questions that follow in the space provided.

Maggie Crumb, an 82-year-old female with a history of emphysema, is brought to the Emergi-Center by her niece. The niece became concerned when her aunt did not phone her for 3 days. The niece reports her aunt has been vomiting and has had severe diarrhea for 5 days. She has not eaten and is having difficulty with her speech. The niece says to the nurse, "My aunt looks terrible, she looks very thin to me. She must be dehydrated. I know she is not a big lady and weighs about 110 pounds—but now, I just do not know." Maggie Crumb responds with the statement, "I am so tired; it's an effort to do anything. I feel very weak. I do not think my legs will hold me up."

1. Write five focused interview questions the nurse should ask this client or the niece.

   1.

   2.

   3.

   4.

   5.

2. The nurse begins the physical assessment by performing a rapid assessment. What data should the nurse gather?

3. Identify the anticipated findings for each of the following as the nurse proceeds with the physical assessment. Place your response on the line provided. Utilize previous chapter information as needed.

   1. Skin turgor _____   **5.** Serum sodium _____

   2. Skin color _____   **6.** Level of consciousness _____

   3. Mucous membranes _____   **7.** Behavior _____

   4. Weight _____   **8.** Serum potassium _____

   The primary care provider makes a diagnosis of acute gastroenteritis with dehydration (hyperosmolar imbalance). It is decided the client needs to stay at the center to initiate fluid replacement.

4. Write one short-term goal for this client.

5. Write two nursing interventions for this client.

   1.

   2.

6. Describe a projected means for evaluation.

TYPES OF ASSESSMENT

1. Name two assessment types the nurse will perform when assessing a client in the hospital setting.

   1.

   2.

2. Read each client situation below and decide which type of assessment will be used by the nurse. On each line provided, place an "R" for rapid assessment or an "I" for initial or routine assessment.

_____ 1. A 5-year-old boy comes to the clinic with his mother to obtain health clearance for kindergarten registration.

_____ 2. A 70-year-old has a 30 mmHg systolic BP drop in the postanesthesia room.

_____ 3. A night nurse begins shift rounds at 12:15 a.m. following shift report.

_____ 4. An LPN takes the BP of her client prior to giving an antihypertensive medication.

_____ 5. A 22-year-old female visits her healthcare provider to seek confirmation of pregnancy.

_____ 6. A 16-year-old cheerleader begins to wheeze during practice and reports to the school nurse.

_____ 7. A 29-year-old female returns to the postpartum unit following a cesarean section.

_____ 8. A CNA in the long-term care agency monitors the oral intake of five clients daily.

3. Place the following nursing activities for the rapid assessment in proper sequential order from 1 through 6.

_____ Observe for signs of distress.

_____ Enter the room.

_____ Wash your hands.

_____ Note the location of the client.

_____ Introduce yourself.

_____ Ask the client his or her name.

4. The nurse has entered a client's room and will complete a rapid assessment. Review the figures below and identify nursing actions and nursing observations. You should have at least 10 responses.

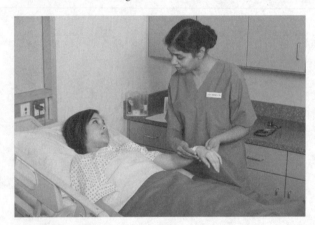 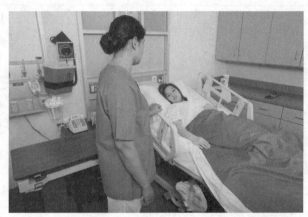

1.

2.

3.

4.

5.

6.

7.

8.

9.

10.

5. The primary nurse is discussing the nursing care of a client with the student nurse assigned to this client.

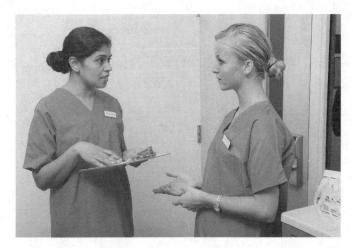

The nurse tells the student: "The client was medicated 3 hours and 45 minutes ago. She just told me she is having pain." The primary nurse instructs the student to complete a pain assessment and then they will initiate nursing interventions based on the assessment findings.

1. How will the student nurse conduct a pain assessment?

2. The assessment indicates incisional pain of 7 on a scale of 0 to 10. You, as the student, give the pain medication as ordered. What is required at this time?

EXPECTED FINDINGS FOR A RESPIRATORY ASSESSMENT ACROSS THE AGE SPAN

Answer the following questions regarding assessment of the respiratory status of a client. Refer to Chapter 17.

1. Before entering a client's room to assess the respiratory status, you identify common factors to be assessed in all clients across the age span. Name seven common factors.

   1. _____
   2. _____
   3. _____
   4. _____
   5. _____
   6. _____
   7. _____

2. Match the expected findings of the respiratory rate per minute with the following age groups.

   Newborn _____ 12–20 per minute   Young adult _____ 30–80 per minute

   School-age child _____ 20–30 per minute   Older adult _____ 15–25 per minute

3. Identify five behaviors you anticipate finding when you assess the respiratory effort of the newborn.

   1.

   2.

   3.

   4.

   5.

4. Identify four behaviors you expect to find when performing a respiratory assessment on a child.

   1.

   2.

   3.

   4.

5. Identify four expected respiratory findings in an adult.

   1.

   2.

   3.

   4.

APPLICATION OF THE CRITICAL THINKING PROCESS

Read the scenario below and then answer the questions that follow in the space provided.

> You are taking report from the night nurse, and the CNA comes to you to report that a client in room 3020A is having trouble breathing. Having received report, you know his name, age, and medical diagnosis, and the surgical procedure performed on his left leg the day before. You immediately leave and go to the bedside of the client.

1. What type of assessment will you perform?

2. How will you confirm the identity of the client?

3. Identify five specific client behaviors that you will assess.

   1.

   2.

   3.

   4.

   5.

4. What additional information is needed? Provide a rationale.

NURSING ASSESSMENT

Review the figure below and list the nursing observations.

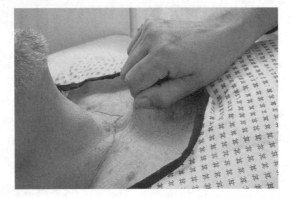

1. What is the nurse doing in this picture?

2. Is the technique correct?

3. If yes, proceed. If no, give the nurse direction to correct her technique.

4. What are the anticipated normal findings?

5. What other parts of the body could be used?

6. List variations in findings. Relate to client condition (e.g., tenting = dehydration, elevated temperature, aging population, etc.).

7. If the skin returns immediately, how will the nurse chart this?

ASSESSMENT AND DOCUMENTATION

Perform a hospitalized client assessment on your lab partner utilizing the skills lab equipment on campus. Assessment data may be fabricated. Document your findings on the following documentation form.

Note: NPSG = National Patient Safety Goals incorporated into care.

Rapid Assessment

Requires 1 minute or less to complete.

Collected data used to prioritize nursing actions and interventions.

Perform hand hygiene (NPSG.07.01.01).

Note isolation precautions, latex allergies, or fall precautions.

Enter the room.

Identify yourself and explain that you will be providing care for a given time period.

Ask the patient's name and identify the patient using at least two patient identifiers, such as wristband and identification number (NPSG.01.01.01).

Note the location of the patient (bed, chair, bathroom).

If in bed, is it in the lowest position and is the call bell in reach?

Observe for level of consciousness.

Observe for signs of distress.

Observe skin color and respiratory effort.

Observe posture, facial expression, and symmetry.

Observe the patient's response to your introduction.

Observe speech for clarity.

Place a hand on the patient and assess skin temperature.

Note any equipment that is immediately visible.

Explain that you will return shortly.

Discuss with the faculty, preceptor, or staff, as needed.

Document findings.

Routine or Initial Assessment

1. Introduction

Perform hand hygiene (NPSG 07.01.01).

Enter the room.

Identify yourself and explain that you will be providing care for a given length of time.

Ask the patient's name and identify the patient using at least two patient identifiers, such as wristband and identification number (NPSG 01.01.01).

Note the patient's location (bed, chair, bathroom).

Note that call bell is in reach.

2. General Appearance

Observe the following:

Level of consciousness

Respiratory status

Skin color

Nutritional status

Facial expression—symmetry and appropriateness

Body posture and position; relaxation, comfort, or pain

Clarity, fluency, quality, and appropriateness of speech

Hygiene and grooming

Response to your introduction in relation to hearing and congruence with situation

3. Measurement

Temperature

Pulses—radial, dorsalis pedis bilaterally

Respirations

Blood pressure (bilaterally if not contraindicated)

Pain—use of rating scale. Correlate with administration of pain medication if so indicated (NPSG.03.06.01).

Pulse oximetry

4. Respiratory System

Respiratory effort

Oxygen therapy—mask, nasal cannula; check placement and flow meter (NPSG.06.01.01).

Auscultate breath sounds—posterior and anterior.

Seek assistance for positioning if required.

Assess for coughing; if productive, assess sputum.

5. Cardiovascular System

Auscultate apical pulse for rate and rhythm.

Assess heart sounds in five auscultatory areas.

Assess for capillary refill.

Assess for peripheral edema.

Assess intravenous (IV) site (NPSG.07.04.01), and if IV fluid is running, verify that it is the correct solution and rate (NPSG.03.06.01).

6. Abdomen

Inspect for contour, skin color, and pulsations.

Auscultate bowel sounds.

Palpate and percuss.

Assess the time of the most recent bowel elimination and/or flatus.

Assess drains, tubes, dressings when indicated (NPSG.07.05.01).

7. Genitourinary

Assess urine output—voiding—frequency and amount, or catheter drainage amount (NPSG.07.06.01).

Assess the color and clarity of urine.

8. Skin

Palpate skin temperature, moisture.

Assess skin turgor.

Assess for lesions.

Assess wounds and incision lines if present (NPSG.07.05.01).

Utilize standardized tools to determine risk for skin problems (scales/questionnaires).

Assess functioning of any devices applied on the skin or used to prevent pressure.

9. Activity

Assess symmetry and coordination of movements throughout the assessment.

Assess the ability to move self to sitting and standing positions.

Assess for presence of and use of assistive devices.

Use standardized measures to evaluate risk for falls.

Assess the environment for hazards related to mobility.

10. Documentation

Discuss with the faculty, preceptor, or staff, as needed.

Document findings according to agency policy.

NCLEX®-STYLE REVIEW QUESTIONS

Read each question carefully. Choose the best answer for each question.

1. A nurse receives report on a hospitalized client 6 hours after a major abdominal surgery. On initial assessment of the client, the nurse notices that the surgical dressing is covered in bright red blood. What is the nurse's initial action?
   1. Inform the healthcare provider immediately
   2. Assess vital signs of the client
   3. Transfuse the client with 2 units of blood
   4. Call another nurse to confirm

2. A hospitalized client complains of severe headaches and states that he experiences headaches only when his blood pressure is high. What is the appropriate response of the nurse caring for this client?
   1. "Don't worry; your blood pressure was normal an hour ago"
   2. "I will give you medication for your headache"
   3. "Let me check your blood pressure and see what it is"
   4. "Your headache is part of the disease process"

3. An elderly client's family member reports that the client is depressed after being admitted to the hospital and has lost all motivation to live. The family also reports that the client was very active at home prior to hospital admission. What is the nurse's best action?
   1. Tell the family that everything will be all right
   2. Contact the primary healthcare provider and report the situation
   3. Make the family understand that all clients get depressed during hospitalization
   4. Ask the family member to leave the client alone to rest

4. A nurse administering medications to a client notices that the client has many visitors, including children, in the room. The client refuses to take the medications when the visitors are present and requests that the nurse leave the medication at the bedside. What is the nurse's best response?
   1. "Sure, no problem! You know what you are doing"
   2. To document that the client refused medications
   3. "I will bring the medications back when the visitors leave"
   4. "If you can take these children out of the room, I will leave the medications"

5. Nurses routinely assess all assigned clients and document the findings within a reasonable time of the beginning of the shift. The hospital policy states that all clients must be assessed at the beginning of each shift. A new nurse on the unit assesses one of the clients 2 hours after the beginning of the shift because the nurse was busy with another ill client. Which of the following actions of a new graduate nurse is not acceptable?
   1. Document for the beginning of the shift
   2. Document the time the assessment was done
   3. Report to the charge nurse
   4. Request help at the beginning of the shift

29 The Complete Health Assessment

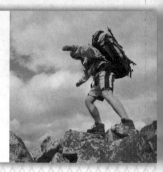

Many of the great achievements of the world were accomplished by tired and discouraged men who kept on working.

—Unknown

This chapter is designed to help the student integrate all the information learned in order to be successful when conducting a complete health assessment.

OBJECTIVES

At the completion of these exercises, you will be able to:

1. Define terms related to health and assessment.
2. Describe the elements of a complete health assessment.
3. Describe communication techniques.
4. Describe the components of the client interview.
5. Apply the concepts of the communication process.
6. Describe the sources of information used by the nurse to obtain client data.
7. Apply client data to the components of the health history.
8. Write focused interview questions related to the complete health assessment.
9. Identify expected findings from the assessment of the integumentary system in selected age groups.
10. Categorize assessment techniques and findings by systems.
11. Apply critical thinking in analysis of a case study.
12. Conduct a complete health assessment on a laboratory partner.
13. Document a complete health assessment.
14. Respond to NCLEX®-style questions related to the complete health assessment.

HEALTH ASSESSMENT

Key Terms

Define the following terms.

1. Health

2. Wellness

3. Illness

4. Comprehensive health assessment

Characteristics

1. Identify three component parts of the comprehensive health assessment.

   1.

   2.

   3.

2. Identify the type of data collected by the nurse when obtaining data for each of the component parts of a complete health assessment.

   1.

   2.

   3.

COMMUNICATION

Therapeutic Communication

Explain how therapeutic communication techniques will be helpful throughout nursing practice.

Interview

1. Define the interview process.

2. List the three phases of the interview process.

   1.

   2.

   3.

3. Indicate when each of the phases is used by the nurse.

Techniques

Describe the following techniques and provide an example of each. Indicate by circling if the example will enhance or hinder the communication process.

1. Attending _____

   Example _____

   Enhance   Hinder

2. Paraphrasing _____

   Example _____

   Enhance   Hinder

3. Use of medical and technical terms _____

   Example _____

   Enhance   Hinder

4. Focusing _____

   Example _____

   Enhance   Hinder

5. Passing judgment _____

   Example _____

   Enhance   Hinder

6. Reflecting _____

   Example _____

   Enhance   Hinder

7. False reassurance _____

   Example _____

   Enhance   Hinder

8. Summarizing _____

   Example _____

   Enhance   Hinder

9. Direct leading _____

   Example _____

   Enhance   Hinder

10. Questioning _____

    Example _____

    Enhance   Hinder

FOCUSED INTERVIEW

Read the scenario below and then answer the questions that follow in the space provided.

A middle-age adult male is married and has two school-age sons. He works as a department supervisor in the office of a large construction firm and is a busy family man. His father died when he was in high school and now his paternal uncle is in the hospital for a myocardial infarction (commonly known as a heart attack). His cousin, who is 2 years older than him, has coronary artery disease. Because he is overweight and has an elevated cholesterol level and a stressful job, he decides to visit the nurse practitioner in the Health and Wellness Center at work. The following is an excerpt from the focused interview between the nurse and this client.

Nurse: "Good afternoon. What brings you here today?"

Client: "I'm concerned. My uncle is in the hospital with a heart attack. His son, my cousin, also has heart problems. I'm afraid I might be next. My doctor told me my cholesterol level is high. I'm not sure what that means."

Nurse: "You seem to be concerned."

Client: "Yes, I am. I have two young sons and a wife, and I need to keep working. I can't afford any health problems."

Nurse: "Well, if you would lose 30 or more pounds your cholesterol level will drop and you would have nothing to worry about." (This is said with a sharp tone of voice.)

Client: "Oh!"

1. Review the first statement made by the nurse.

   a. What technique is the nurse using?

   b. Will this enhance or hinder the communication process?

   c. Provide a rationale for your decision.

2. Review the second statement made by the nurse.

   a. What technique is the nurse using?

   b. Will this technique encourage or hinder the communication process?

   c. Provide a rationale for your decision.

   d. Is there a need for the nurse to use a different strategy?

3. Review the third statement made by the nurse.

   a. Identify the three strategies used by the nurse in this statement.
      1.

      2.

      3.

   b. Do these strategies encourage the communication process?
      1.

      2.

      3.

4. Write three focused interview questions that the nurse could use that would enhance the communication process.
   1.
   2.
   3.

SOURCE OF INFORMATION

1. Define the sources of information used by the nurse to obtain client data.

   1. Primary source:

   2. Secondary source:

2. Read the following list of data obtained by the nurse. Identify each piece of data as primary or secondary by writing a "P" for primary or an "S" for secondary.

   _____ 1. "My leg hurts"

   _____ 2. Seems to have trouble breathing

   _____ 3. Complete blood count within normal limits

   _____ 4. "I am always tired"

   _____ 5. BP 156/90

   _____ 6. Recorded urinary output of 300 ml

HEALTH HISTORY

1. Match the client data found in Column A with the component part of the health history in Column B by placing the letter or letters on each line provided. The component part might be used once, more than once, or not at all.

Column A Client Data

_____ 1. African American

_____ 2. Presence of yellow phlegm

_____ 3. MMR 3 months ago

_____ 4. Appendectomy age 7

_____ 5. Father died of MI

_____ 6. High school diploma

_____ 7. Young adult

_____ 8. No current health complaints

_____ 9. Exercises 3 times/week

_____ 10. Eats breakfast daily

_____ 11. Menstrual period every 28 days

_____ 12. Sister has asthma

_____ 13. Has trouble breathing when lying down

_____ 14. Can distinguish odors

Column B Component Part

A. Review of Systems

B. Biographical Data

C. Family History

D. Medical History

E. Surgical History

F. Current Health Status

G. Psychosocial Data

FOCUSED INTERVIEW QUESTIONS

Write four focused interview questions you would use for each given topic and age.

1. Older adult: activities of daily living (ADLs)

   1. _____

   2. _____

   3. _____

   4. _____

2. School-age child: A 7-year-old falls on the playground at school and comes to the school nurse crying and with blood on his shirt.

   1. _____

   2. _____

   3. _____

   4. _____

EXPECTED FINDINGS

For each of the selected age groups, identify expected physical assessment findings for the assessment of the skin, hair, and nails.

1. Newborn

   1. _____

   2. _____

   3. _____

   4. _____

   5. _____

2. Child

1. _____

2. _____

3. _____

3. Pregnant female

1. _____

2. _____

3. _____

4. Adult

1. _____

2. _____

3. _____

4. _____

5. Older adult: Describe the anticipated physical assessment findings of the skin regarding:

1. Turgor: _____

2. Moisture: _____

3. Texture: _____

4. Color: _____

5. Temperature: _____

BODY SYSTEMS

Match the assessment technique in Column A with the body system found in Column B. The body system may be used once, more than once, or not at all.

<u>Column A</u>

_____ 1. Apical pulse 68

_____ 2. Turgor resilient

_____ 3. Palpation of Skene's glands

_____ 4. Diaphragmatic excursion

_____ 5. Romberg test positive

_____ 6. Capillary refill

_____ 7. Phalen's test

_____ 8. Palpating the spleen

_____ 9. Confrontation test

_____ 10. Babinski test

_____ 11. Tactile fremitus

_____ 12. Tinel's sign

_____ 13. Palpating the tragus

_____ 14. Ability to calculate

_____ 15. CVA tenderness

_____ 16. Rebound tenderness

_____ 17. Whisper pectoriloquy

_____ 18. Whisper test

_____ 19. Cardinal fields

_____ 20. Palpation of the axillae

<u>Column B</u>

A. Skin, hair, nails

B. Head, neck, and related lymphatics

C. Eye

D. Ear, nose, mouth, throat

E. Respiratory

F. Breast and axillae

G. Cardiovascular

H. Peripheral vascular

I. Abdomen

J. Urinary

K. Male reproductive

L. Female reproductive

M. Musculoskeletal

N. Neurologic

APPLICATION OF THE CRITICAL THINKING PROCESS

Read the scenario below and then answer the questions that follow in the space provided.

> A middle-aged male reports to the healthcare provider's office for his yearly physical examination. He is 55 years old and has done the same type of job for the past 25 years. The company is going through an economic crisis, and the client is concerned about losing his job. He reports to the nurse, "I feel healthy except for occasional heartburn or pressure right here (pointing to the left side of his chest), and sometimes I feel my heart racing." The following is an excerpt from the focused interview between the nurse and this client:

Nurse: "Good morning! I see that you were here last year for your physical."

Client: "Yes, that is correct."

Nurse: "Tell me how your health has been the past year."

Client: "I consider myself a really healthy person. I haven't been out sick from work all year. It is just the pressure that I get right here." (Again, the client points to the left side of his chest.)

Nurse: "Tell me more about this heartburn and the pressure on your chest."

Client: "It is just here, and not all the time."

Nurse: "Does the heartburn and pressure get worse before or after you eat?"

Client: "I have not noticed any change when I eat."

Nurse: "When do you notice the change?"

Client: "When I am at work either during or after our management meetings."

1. Based on the information obtained from the client, what subjective data could be the contributing factor for his "pressure in the chest area"?

2. When interviewing the client, what familial tendencies should be included in the interview?

3. What medical conditions could contribute to the client's risk of heart disease?

4. What other questions would be helpful to the nurse regarding the type of pain the client is experiencing?

5. How would you proceed with the physical assessment of the client?

ASSESSMENT AND DOCUMENTATION

Perform a complete health assessment on your lab partner and document your findings on the following documentation form.

Name:_____Date:_____

Age: _____ Gender: _____

Reason for today's visit _____

_____

THE HEALTH HISTORY

The health history would include all areas of the cultural and spiritual assessment, noted in previous chapters.

For a child, ask about the child's grade level and school _____

Document data as subjective data.

APPEARANCE AND MENTAL STATUS

Compare stated age with appearance. Does chronological age match developmental age? If not, document

observations _____

_____

Assess level of consciousness—alert to person, place, time? _____

_____

Does client's body build, height, and weight match to chronological age? _____

_____

Does client's body build, height, and weight affect the client's lifestyle and health? _____

_____

Observe client's facial expression, posture, and position for any issues/concerns/abnormalities _____

_____

Observe client's mobility by having the client walk across the room or down the hallway—note gait and any

issues/concerns/abnormalities _____

_____

Observe client's overall hygiene and grooming—body odor, condition of clothes, hair, etc. _____

_____

Note odor of breath _____

Note signs of overall health or illness such as skin color, signs of pain, etc. _____

_____

Assess client's attitude, attentiveness, affect, mood, and appropriateness of responses _____

_____

Assess client's speech by listening for quantity, quality, relevance, and organization of speech _____

_____

Client should change into an examination gown upon completion of this component of the assessment. Privacy should be provided at this time. The client should also have the opportunity to empty his or her bladder and, if necessary, a urine specimen should be collected.

MEASUREMENTS

Height _____ Weight _____ Skinfold thickness _____

Body mass index (BMI) _____

Client vision assessment with Snellen chart, or age-appropriate screening tool for children _____

_____

Client vision assessment with Jaeger card _____

VITAL SIGNS

Assess radial pulses bilaterally (L) _____ (R) _____

Respirations _____ Temperature _____

Blood pressure bilaterally (L) _____ (R) _____

Assess for pain with appropriate pain scale for client's age/developmental status _____

_____

SKIN, HAIR, AND NAILS

Inspect the following areas for color and uniformity of color; palpate the skin temperature and note moisture, turgor, and edema; inspect, palpate, measure, and describe any lesions

Face _____

Neck _____

Upper extremities _____

Lower extremities _____

Inspect the hair on the body and scalp; palpate hair for texture and moisture _____

_____

Inspect the fingernails for curvature, angle, and color _____

_____

Palpate the nails for texture and capillary refill _____

_____

HEAD, NECK, AND RELATED LYMPHATICS

Inspect the skull for size, shape, and symmetry _____

_____

Observe facial expressions and symmetry of facial features and movements (cranial nerves V and VII)

_____

_____

Palpate the skull and lymph nodes of the head and neck _____

_____

Palpate the muscles of the face (cranial nerve V) _____

Assess facial response to sensory stimulation (cranial nerve V) _____

Inspect the neck for symmetry, pulsations, swelling, or masses _____

_____

Assess range of motion and strength of muscles against resistance. Observe as the client moves the head forward and back and side to side and shrugs the shoulders (cranial nerve XI) _____

_____

Palpate the trachea _____

Palpate the thyroid for symmetry and masses _____

_____

Palpate and auscultate the carotid arteries, one at a time _____

EYES

Inspect the external eye _____

Inspect the pupils for color, size, shape, and equality _____

_____

Test the visual fields (cranial nerve II) _____

Test extraocular movements (cranial nerves III, IV, VI) _____

Test pupillary reaction to light and accommodations (cranial nerve III) _____

Darken the room and use the ophthalmoscope to assess the red reflex, optic disc, retinal vessels, retinal

background, macula, and fovea centralis _____

_____

EARS, NOSE, MOUTH, AND THROAT

Inspect the external ears _____

Palpate the auricle and tragus of each ear _____

Inspect each external ear canal and the tympanic membrane with an otoscope _____

_____

Test hearing in each ear using the whisper, Weber, and Rinne tests (cranial nerve VIII) _____

_____

Assess patency of the nares _____

Test sense of smell (cranial nerve I) _____

Inspect the internal nose with a nasal speculum or otoscope _____

_____

Palpate the nose and sinuses, noting pain, pressure, or sensitivity _____

_____

Palpate the temporal artery _____

Palpate the temporomandibular joint (TMJ) as the client opens and closes the mouth _____

_____

Inspect the lips for color, dryness, fissures, and other abnormalities _____

_____

Use a penlight to inspect the tongue, palates, buccal mucosa, gums, teeth, the opening to the salivary glands,

tonsils, and oropharynx, noting any issues/concerns/abnormalities _____

_____

Test the sense of taste (cranial nerve VII) _____

_____

Palpate the tongue, gums, and floor of the mouth, noting any issues/concerns/abnormalities _____

_____

Observe the uvula for position and mobility as the client says "ah," and test the gag reflex (cranial nerves IX, X)

_____

_____

Observe as the client protrudes the tongue, noting any issues/concerns/abnormalities (cranial nerve XII)

_____

THE RESPIRATORY SYSTEM, BREASTS, AND AXILLAE

Inspect the skin of the posterior chest, noting color, uniformity of color, skin temperature, moisture, turgor, and edema _____

_____

Inspect the posterior chest for symmetry, musculoskeletal development, and thoracic configuration

_____

_____

Observe respiratory excursion/effort of the client _____

_____

Auscultate posterior lung sounds _____

Palpate and percuss the costovertebral angle for tenderness _____

_____

Palpate for thoracic expansion and tactile fremitus _____

_____

Inspect and palpate the scapula and spine _____

Percuss the posterior thorax _____

Percuss for diaphragmatic excursion _____

Inspect the skin of the anterior chest, noting color, uniformity of color, skin temperature, moisture, turgor, and edema _____

_____

Assess range of motion and movement against resistance of the upper extremities _____

_____

Inspect the breast for symmetry, mobility, masses, dimpling, and nipple retraction; ask the post-pubescent female to lift arms over her head, press her hands on her hips, and lean forward as you inspect

_____

Auscultate anterior lung sounds _____

Palpate the axillary, supraclavicular, and infraclavicular lymph nodes _____

_____

Palpate the breasts and nipples _____

Palpate the anterior chest _____

Percuss the anterior thorax _____

THE CARDIOVASCULAR SYSTEM

Inspect the neck for jugular pulsations or distention _____

_____

Inspect and palpate the chest for pulsations, lifts, or heaves _____

_____

Use the bell and diaphragm of the stethoscope to auscultate for heart sounds _____

_____

At each area of auscultation, distinguish the rate, rhythm, and location of S1 and S2 _____

_____

Palpate the apical pulse and note the intensity and location _____

_____

THE ABDOMEN

Inspect the skin of the abdomen _____

_____

Inspect the abdomen for symmetry, contour, movement, and pulsation _____

_____

Auscultate the abdomen for bowel sounds _____

_____

Auscultate the abdomen for vascular sounds _____

_____

Palpate the liver, spleen, and kidneys _____

_____

Palpate to determine if tenderness, masses, or distention is present _____

_____

Palpate the inguinal region for pulses, lymph nodes, and presence of hernias _____

_____

Percuss the abdomen in all quadrants _____

Percuss the abdomen to determine liver and spleen size _____

_____

THE MUSCULOSKELETAL SYSTEM

Test range of motion and strength in the hips, knees, ankles, and feet _____

_____

_____

_____

Assist the client to a standing position and inspect the skin of the posterior legs _____

_____

Perform the Romberg test _____

_____

Observe as the client walks in a natural gait _____

Observe the client walking heel to toe _____

Observe the client stand on the right foot, then the left foot with eyes closed _____

_____

Observe as the client performs a shallow knee bend _____

Stand behind the client and observe the spine as the client touches the toes _____

_____

Test range of motion of the spine _____

THE NEUROLOGIC SYSTEM

Assess sensory function—include light touch, tactile location, pain, temperature, vibratory sense, kinesthetic sensation, and tactile discrimination _____

_____

Test position sense _____

Test cerebellar function with finger-to-nose test _____

Test cerebellar function with heel-shin test _____

Test stereognosis and graphesthesia _____

Test tendon reflexes bilaterally and compare to chronological/developmental age _____

_____

THE FEMALE REPRODUCTIVE SYSTEM

This system would be assessed as age appropriate for the female client.

Inspect the amount, distribution, and characteristics of pubic hair _____

_____

Inspect the clitoris, urethral orifice, and vaginal orifice _____

_____

Palpate Bartholin's glands _____

Assess the integrity of the pelvic musculature _____

Insert a speculum and examine the internal genitalia _____

_____

Inspect the cervix for shape of the os, color, size, and position _____

_____

For post-pubescent females, obtain a specimen for a Papanicolaou smear _____

_____

Inspect the vaginal walls _____

Perform a bimanual examination _____

Palpate the rectum and rectovaginal walls _____

Observe and test stool for occult blood _____

THE MALE REPRODUCTIVE SYSTEM

This system would be assessed as age appropriate for the male client.

Observe the amount, distribution, and characteristics of pubic hair _____

_____

Inspect the penile shaft, glans, and urethral meatus _____

Observe the color and position of the urethral meatus _____

Inspect the scrotum for appearance, size, and symmetry _____

Palpate the scrotum, testicles, epididymis, and spermatic cord; if a mass is present, then inspect by transil-

lumination _____

Inspect the sacrococcygeal and perianal areas _____

Palpate the rectal walls and prostate gland _____

Observe any stool and test for occult blood _____

Document findings from the comprehensive health assessment according to agency policy. Include all concepts of client safety, standard precautions, and professional standards in the documentation of assessment data. Documentation is important; the data documented from the complete assessment establish a baseline for ongoing client interaction and care.

NCLEX®-STYLE REVIEW QUESTIONS

Read each question carefully. Choose the best answer for each question.

1. The mother of a 12-month-old child tells the nurse, "I can see his belly rumbling. Is this normal?" Which of the following is the best response from the nurse?
    1. "You need to take him to a good pediatric gastroenterologist."
    2. "This means that the gallbladder is digesting fats."
    3. "No—this is not normal."
    4. "The muscles of the abdomen are thin in babies, so you will see this."

2. The client asks the nurse, "Is it normal to have a stomachache almost every day?" Which of the following would be the nurse's best response to this client?
    1. "That's not good at all."
    2. "I would suggest that you see a specialist."
    3. "No one can have a stomachache every day."
    4. "Maybe we can talk about your diet."

3. A 14-year-old male client expresses concern over his "misshaped private parts." Upon examination, the nurse learns the client is concerned about his scrotum. Which of the following would the nurse explain to this client?
    1. "You are right; the testicles should be even."
    2. "This is completely normal."
    3. "I think you should see a specialist."
    4. "Well, your left testicle is lower than your right."

4. A client with a head injury is demonstrating difficulty swallowing and talking. Which cranial nerve would be adversely affected with this head injury?
    1. Glossopharyngeal
    2. Vagus
    3. Hypoglossal
    4. Accessory

5. A client is recovering from a cardiac catheterization during which the right femoral artery was accessed. Which of the following pulses can the nurse use to assess the patency of this artery?
   1. Brachial
   2. Radial
   3. Posterior tibial
   4. Ulnar

6. The nurse hears a heart sound right before S1 on an 80-year-old male client. What can this finding suggest to the nurse?
   1. Nothing; this is normal
   2. This is an atrial gallop and can mean that something is wrong
   3. This is an atrial kick and helps the heart beat better
   4. This is a ventricular gallop and is heard in healthy people

7. An elderly client wants to know when she can stop doing breast exams. What can the nurse say to this client?
   1. "You should have stopped right after menopause."
   2. "You can probably stop in a month or two."
   3. "Breast cancer can still develop when you get older."
   4. "It is not recommended at your age."

8. While teaching, the nurse instructs a client about immunizations. What level of prevention does immunizations fall into?
   1. Tertiary
   2. Secondary
   3. Restorative
   4. Primary

9. After completing the health history on a client during assessment, the nurse begins to ask more questions about specific information. What is this portion of the health assessment called?
   1. Documentation follow-up
   2. Focused interview
   3. Physical assessment
   4. Interpretation of findings

10. A nurse is observed talking rudely to a client of a non-American culture. When approached about this behavior, the nurse responds, "These people have no right to be in the United States." What is the nurse demonstrating?
    1. Material culture
    2. Nonmaterial culture
    3. Competent cultural care
    4. Ethnocentrism